T0054324

MASSAGE FOR COUPLES

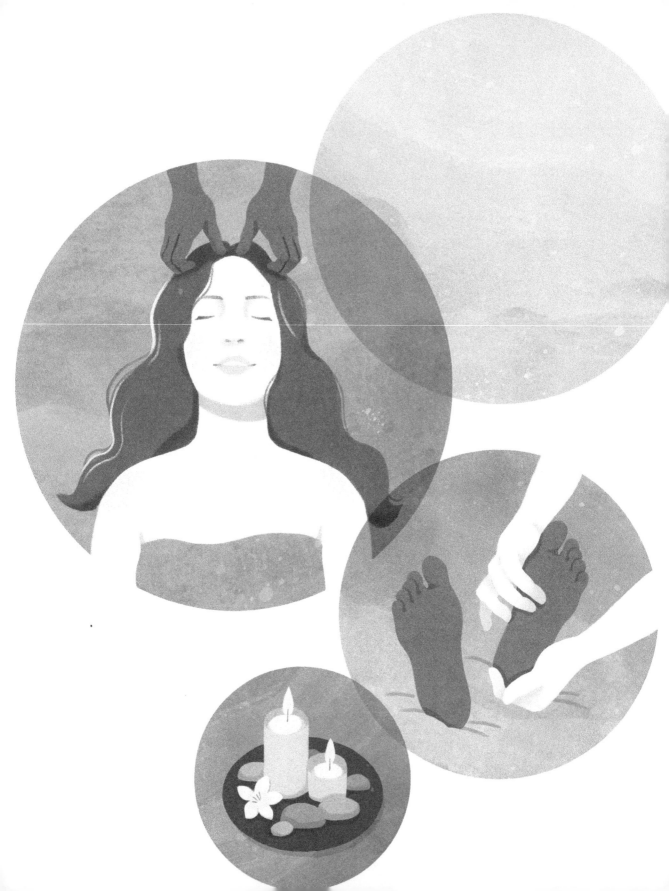

MASSAGE
for Couples

Heal, Soothe, and Connect with the One You Love

Ashley Dwyer, LMT

ROCKRIDGE PRESS

Copyright © 2020 by Rockridge Press, Emeryville, California

No part of this publication may be reproduced, stored in a retrieval system, or transmitted in any form or by any means, electronic, mechanical, photocopying, recording, scanning, or otherwise, except as permitted under Sections 107 or 108 of the 1976 United States Copyright Act, without the prior written permission of the Publisher. Requests to the Publisher for permission should be addressed to the Permissions Department, Rockridge Press, 6005 Shellmound Street, Suite 175, Emeryville, CA 94608.

Limit of Liability/Disclaimer of Warranty: The Publisher and the author make no representations or warranties with respect to the accuracy or completeness of the contents of this work and specifically disclaim all warranties, including without limitation warranties of fitness for a particular purpose. No warranty may be created or extended by sales or promotional materials. The advice and strategies contained herein may not be suitable for every situation. This work is sold with the understanding that the Publisher is not engaged in rendering medical, legal, or other professional advice or services. If professional assistance is required, the services of a competent professional person should be sought. Neither the Publisher nor the author shall be liable for damages arising herefrom. The fact that an individual, organization, or website is referred to in this work as a citation and/or potential source of further information does not mean that the author or the Publisher endorses the information the individual, organization, or website may provide or recommendations they/it may make. Further, readers should be aware that websites listed in this work may have changed or disappeared between when this work was written and when it is read.

For general information on our other products and services or to obtain technical support, please contact our Customer Care Department within the United States at (866) 744-2665, or outside the United States at (510) 253-0500.

Rockridge Press publishes its books in a variety of electronic and print formats. Some content that appears in print may not be available in electronic books, and vice versa.

TRADEMARKS: Rockridge Press and the Rockridge Press logo are trademarks or registered trademarks of Callisto Media Inc. and/or its affiliates, in the United States and other countries, and may not be used without written permission. All other trademarks are the property of their respective owners. Rockridge Press is not associated with any product or vendor mentioned in this book.

Interior and Cover Designer: Tricia Jang
Art Producer: Hannah Dickerson
Editor: Rochelle Torke
Production Manager: Giraud Lorber
Production Editor: Sigi Nacson

Illustrations © 2020 Christy Ni
Author photo courtesy of Laura Tompkins/Laura Belle Photography

ISBN: Print 978-1-64611-869-4 | eBook 978-1-64611-870-0

R1

This book is for home and personal use only. It's not intended to treat or diagnose a medical condition or replace regular medical or psychiatric care. It doesn't replace formal massage training or prepare readers for the licensing board exam. Please check your local and state guidelines for further laws, regulations, and information pertaining to massage therapy.

To my son, Skyler, my loyal staff, clients, and students at Fire & Ice Therapeutic Massage and the Massage Innovation Network for Therapists. Thank you for believing in me.

Contents

Introduction

Many of my clients have asked me for tips on giving better massages to help their partner with aches and pains. Sometimes they're intimidated by massage or have decided that they're "just not good at it." Some say massage hurts their hands or they're not sure about using the right pressure.

Learning to massage another human can be tricky at first, but I'm here to tell you that it's a skill you can learn and enjoy. For example, the first person I massaged in school nearly kicked me because he was extremely ticklish and it was hard to find the right amount of pressure to suit him.

Practice makes perfect, though. After many years of working with this healing art, and over five years as a professional massage therapist, I can find all kinds of things under the skin with my eyes open or closed. I help people ease their pain from a holistic standpoint and gain relief from stress and fatigue. I have also taught a couples massage class for people who want to support their partners' well-being and enjoy a healthy, enriching way to spend quality time together.

My massage practice, Fire & Ice Therapeutic Massage, was voted "best massage" by North Carolina's *Matthews–Mint Hill Weekly* in 2019. I was nominated for Charlotte Media Group's Small Businessperson of the Year that same year. I did a short series on MindBodyRadio in January 2020 about massage and bodywork where I answered questions from callers about massage. In addition, I have gone on to become an approved continuing education provider, received my certifications in life, business, relationship, and mind-set coaching, and recently completed my business consulting certification.

I own a second business called the Massage Innovation Network for Therapists that provides continuing education for massage therapists. I teach them new techniques beyond the basics of what they learn in school and coach them toward brighter, longer careers.

Whether you are in a new relationship or have been in a marriage for decades, I encourage you to read through this book in its entirety. The knowledge and background information you'll gain—including some light biology and anatomy lessons—will help you refine your skills and give truly transformative, bliss-inspiring massages. This book can also prepare you for a closer, more nurturing and intimate relationship with the one you love.

How to Use This Book

The goal of this book is to help you grow in your relationship and in your health by sharing massage with your partner. The first part of this book will help you gain confidence in using your hands to provide healing touch. It will help you understand why massage may be beneficial to your budding relationship. As you begin to grow more sensitive to your partner's needs corresponding to touch, I hope that you will find a deeper level of connection. The second part of this book will teach you techniques from Eastern and Western traditions around the world, as well as how to strengthen and develop the skills you have in your own set of hands. The last part of the book will guide you through the body to prepare you to perform massage sequences for special situations and circumstances.

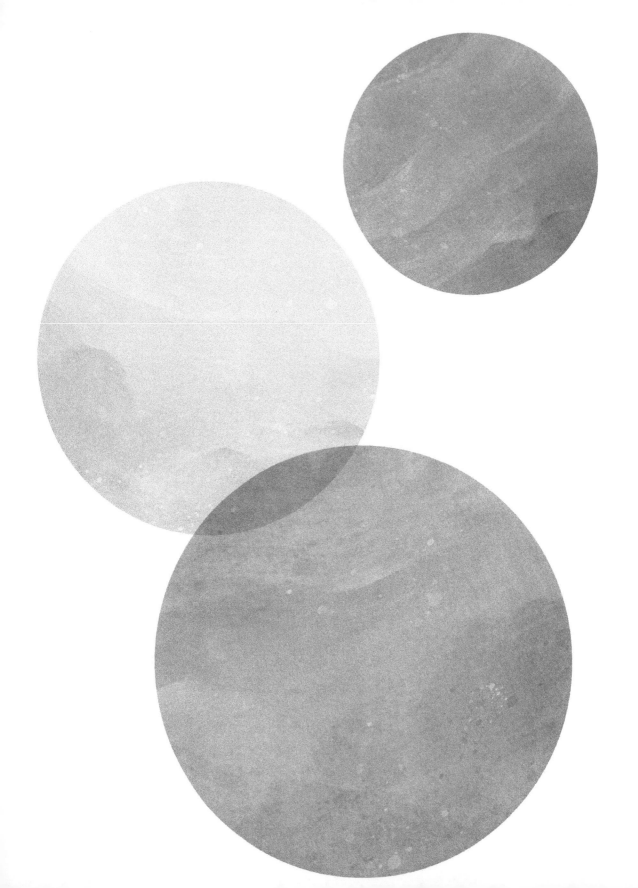

Part 1

THE POWER OF TOUCH

Everyday life can be full of distractions. Couples often spend most of the day apart, and even when they are together they easily fall into domestic busyness. When they do focus on each other, they might talk through their days, sharing the ups and downs, venting, or simply trying to connect to each other through words. Although talking is important, there's another powerful tool for relieving stress and reconnecting with the one you love: soothing touch.

A kind touch can ground the racing mind and bring it into the present moment. Massage is a nourishing practice and a simple, intuitive means for connecting to your partner. It's a way to set time aside to nurture and invest in your relationship, fostering love, trust, patience, intimacy, and health. This book will explain the many benefits of massage and why it can be the perfect way to express caring, affection, and love.

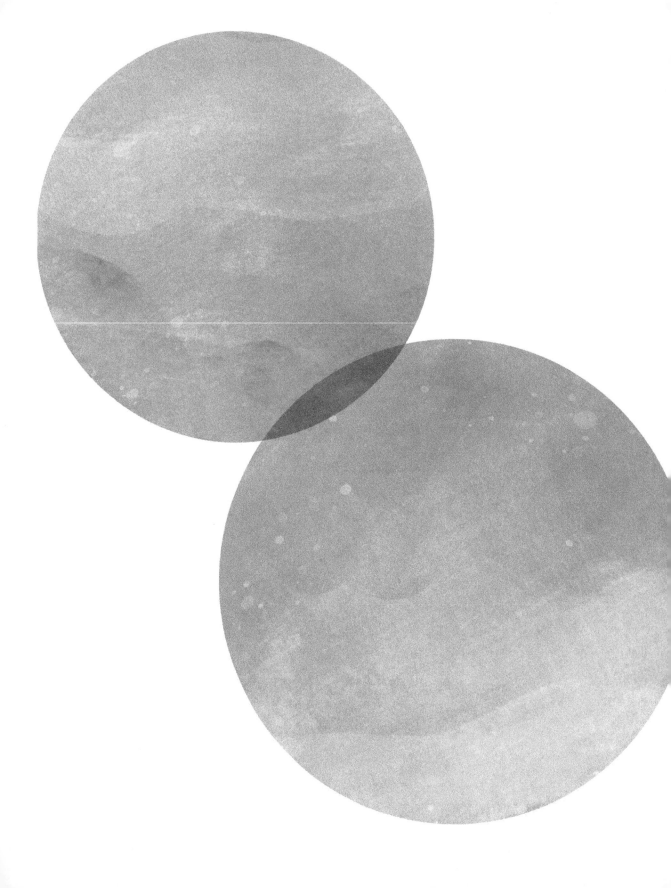

Chapter 1

For Healing, Vitality, and Connection

Touch and massage provide a vast array of benefits providing relief for a variety of ailments, like common tension headaches, sciatic pain, plantar fasciitis, poor circulation, and elevated stress response. The therapeutic massage field has grown tremendously over the last 50 years because people crave the numerous benefits of this healing art. In addition to these health benefits, massage is also a great way to create healthy intimacy in a relationship where the need for touch is undeniable. As a licensed massage and bodywork therapist, I believe that massage belongs in a therapeutic healing environment as well as at home, to be shared with loved ones and partners. In this chapter we will discuss the benefits of touch and how massage therapy at home can help your relationship become sounder, keep you free from illnesses or injuries, and increase strength and energy.

We're Made to Be Touched

From the moment we are born, touch is used to bring circulation into our bodies. A mother pats and rubs her baby's back to soothe them. Small children fall, skin their knees, and we instinctively rub the area to send the pain away. When our stomach hurts, we rub it. This instinctive rubbing response to pain is known as the pain gateway theory. This theory can explain why massage is one of the most ancient, instinctual forms of medicine and is still practiced today. Here are some of its many benefits.

PAIN RELIEF

One of the most undisputed benefits of massage is the increase in circulation. Increasing circulation to an area means bringing blood flow and nutrients to that spot to encourage healing. Closing the "gates" of the pain signal by instinctually massaging the area interrupts the pain pathways sending messages to the brain. This helps reduce the sensation of pain. Nerves do not possess the elastic qualities that muscles have. So when there are underlying adhesions (sometimes called "knots"), the nerve can't move freely through the tissue, resulting in what is sometimes called a nerve impingement. There is also fascia—a thin sheath of fibrous tissue that encloses your muscles and organs and that thickens as we age. Sometimes moving and freeing up the fascia can release an area of restriction and reduce pain. In the case of trigger points, which we will discuss in chapter 3 (page 30), we can release spindle fibers within the muscle that may have prevented the muscle from functioning at its best during stretching and movement.

BRAIN FUNCTION AND HEALTH

During a massage, typically the receiver begins to relax and breathe. When the body relaxes, the mind can spend time processing everything that went on that day, week, or year that it still needs to comprehend. Cortisol, a stress hormone, can cause damage to the brain by creating pathways between the amygdala and the hippocampus, throwing it into a heightened state—known as fight or flight. During fight or flight, in response to stress the body is flooded with hormones that prepare us to flee the scene or fight for our life. Strengthening these responses can have a negative impact on the body, such as anxiety, depression, insomnia, digestive problems, heart disease, weight gain, and memory and concentration issues.

Massage activates the parasympathetic nervous system, which is the opposite of the sympathetic nervous system that includes fight or flight. In this "rest and digest" state, the body relaxes muscles, reduces glandular activity that involves secreting hormones, increases digestion, and lets the brain finally process all of the data that we have been stimulated with over and over again. Then we are able to think more clearly and feel less stressed so we can lead happier, healthier lives.

BONDING TIME

A growing trend in child birthing is skin-to-skin contact, or keeping the baby in direct contact with a parent or loved one. This idea encourages laying the new baby on the skin of its new parents to help their bond grow. One of the benefits of this is self-regulation due to the patterns of the parents' breathing. What if I told you that skin-to-skin contact with your loved one could help you even your breathing and wind down after a stressful day at work or after wrangling children all day?

EMOTIONAL WELL-BEING

Massage from a partner will help you adapt to changes and stressors faster because it's a tangible reminder that we have their love, acceptance, and support. Emotional well-being can be obtained using touch therapies, such as massage. Studies of mammals consistently demonstrate how necessary touch and contact are for developing to adulthood and having a healthy life.

Scientists have recognized that touch is a foundational, physiological, primal need like air, water, food, shelter, clothing, and reproduction. When primal and safety needs have been met, people and animals look for love and belonging, which includes engaging in friendships and intimacy and searching for a sense of connection. These relationship needs lead to self-esteem, respect, status, recognition, strength, and a sense of freedom. A nourishing, healthy relationship involving touch can help achieve each of these requirements for mental and emotional well-being by changing our innate nature for selfishness and self-centeredness through nurturing, building both empathy and the ability to see outside one's own self.

A BETTER NIGHT'S SLEEP

Serotonin levels increase when you receive a massage. This relaxing hormone helps your brain prepare for sleep and encourages the body to produce melatonin, which is essential for regulating the circadian rhythm leading to a good night's sleep. Melatonin also lowers cortisol levels and stimulates the vagus nerve, helping the whole body relax. Additionally, the stimulation of the vagus nerve via massage can increase digestion, making for a healthier appetite.

SKIN HEALTH

The act of massage obviously involves applying a lubricant to the skin. This can help with exfoliation and quicker cell turnover, and even help catch skin diseases (such as skin cancer) early on, when noticing abnormal moles or other anomalies.

IMMUNE SYSTEM

Massage improves immune response by stimulating the lymphatic system, a network of tissues and organs that helps the body remove toxins. Unlike other body systems, the lymph system relies on muscle movements to act as a pump that triggers the flow of lymph—the fluid that carries infection-fighting white blood cells around the body. Massage helps move lymph throughout the body, improving immunity. After exercise, massage can also help reduce areas of soreness by promoting circulation to the affected area.

HORMONES

Touch not only increases circulation, but also helps release hormones throughout the body. Endorphins are feel-good hormones released by the body during a massage. This may help reduce anxiety, depression, and insomnia, leading to a good night's sleep. Oxytocin, which is sometimes referred to as the "cuddling hormone," is released during a massage. This hormone stimulates the parasympathetic nervous system to make the receiver of the massage feel calmer and safer. This can also reduce anxiety and depression. Serotonin levels also increase.

MUSCLE HEALTH

Massage can help release areas of tension, which may reduce headaches, migraines, and other everyday pains. Massage also helps improve range of motion and may prevent arthritis and other joint issues. Muscular tension can also be caused by trauma, which may be held from a strained relationship. If the brain is no longer telling the muscle to contract due to emotional distress, then the muscle can let go and relax.

The History of Massage

The first written descriptions of massage were recorded in China from 3,000 to 5,000 years ago. Massage was incorporated into all aspects of health, using the five elements to heal the body and balance "amma," or energy. Hot and cold stones were used in childbirth and to stop bleeding.

Developed in India, the Ayurvedic healing system also featured early versions of massage. Ayurveda was the first whole-body approach addressing mind, body, and spirit. Still practiced today around the world, Ayurveda focuses on creating harmony throughout the body to avoid "dis-ease" and empower the body to restore itself. The practice supports good health through diet, herbs, oils, and massage.

Egyptians were quite advanced in the use of massage and were the first to value essential oils and practice aromatherapy. Cleopatra received regular baths and massage with jasmine and rose, with sensual effects. Essential oils were a valuable trade commodity.

Many shamanic traditions involve massaging substances into the skin while drumming and chanting to relieve illness. The Hawaiian massage technique lomilomi arose from shamanic tradition and was used primarily to aid in digestion and lovemaking.

Greek and Roman societies used massage for health and pleasure. Herodotus taught Hippocrates the art of rubbing. Hippocrates is known today as the father of medicine. In his writing he described massage, saying: "The physician must be experienced in many things but assuredly also in rubbing [anatripsis]; for things that have the same name have not always the same effects. For rubbing can bind a joint that is too loose and loosen a joint that is too rigid. . . . Rubbing can bind and loosen; can make flesh [referring to the ability to tone muscle tissue] and cause parts to waste [soften and relax]. Hard rubbing binds: soft rubbing loosens; much rubbing causes parts to waste; moderate rubbing makes them grow."

Julius Caesar had massages daily in a society where bathhouses were bountiful. The center of business and pleasure, Rome's bathhouses contained many rooms where patrons not only took baths but were also anointed in oil and massaged, exercised, and had another hot bath before taking a dip in a cold pool.

The history of massage took a turn in the Dark Ages, when European societies began to frown upon touch. Public bathhouses were emptied and nearly disappeared due to the rise of new, proscriptive religious practices.

Physical contact between people in general came under close scrutiny, with many forms of touch declared sinful or overly sensual. The church prohibited massage on Sunday, Wednesday, Friday, the 40 days of Lent, the 40 days before Christmas, and the 3 days prior to communion. Passion, lust, and love itself were heavily scrutinized, as marriage became a social arrangement between families, informed by church guidelines. The church decreed that sex should exist only for producing children. Sexual pleasure was to be avoided by both men and women as it was thought to engender bad behavior and other pathologies. Sex for barren and menopausal women was banned entirely. Couples, the church said, should engage in sex infrequently, and in the missionary position only.

In time, the undeniable health benefits of massage led to the slow resurgence of the healing art. In the early 1800s Peter Ling learned to revitalize soft tissue among gymnasts, using techniques we now call Swedish massage. Johann Metzger later assigned French names to the techniques. In 1884, the Society of Trained Masseuses formed in England to promote the health value of massage. It later became the Chartered Society of Physiotherapy and promoted massage during both world wars.

By the 1950s, professional therapeutic massage was gaining popularity in the United States. By the 1980s, massage became regulated to protect the public, and certification programs became more standardized. The rise of concepts like "mind-body detox" boosted the credibility and validity of massage as a health tool. Today in most US states, massage therapists must pass a certification exam before applying for licensure. However, whereas professional massage therapists offer deep knowledge of massage techniques and human anatomy, novice massage at home still offers tremendous benefit.

Physical Anatomy

Massage can be used on almost any spot on the body. Some areas may be more sensitive than others and require lighter pressure. These areas include the eyes, front of the neck, abdomen, and armpits. Areas with thinner skin are more sensitive to damage and injury. If you ever feel a pulse, then you want to move away from that area to prevent injury. Areas where lymph nodes lie, such as the groin, armpits, and neck, require lighter work to avoid damaging underlying structures.

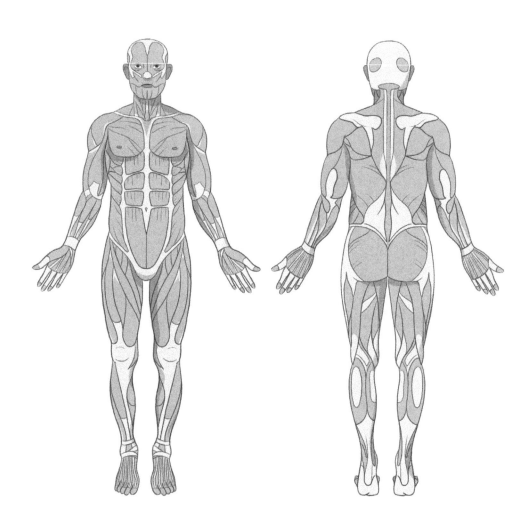

Energy Anatomy

In traditional Chinese medicine, "qi," or life energy, flows through the body across a network referred to as the meridian system. In Ayurveda, this is called "prana." Through this network, life force feeds all areas of the body, including the brain, nervous system, and all organs and tissues. When qi flow to an area is disturbed, blocked, or suppressed, illness or pain in that area will manifest itself. Ancient Taoists practiced a breathing method called "tui na" while doing "qigong" (exercises used to harness and balance energy) to produce healthy, balanced, free-flowing qi. This breathing method expanded the abdomen during inhalation and contracted the abdomen during exhalation to balance the energy within the body.

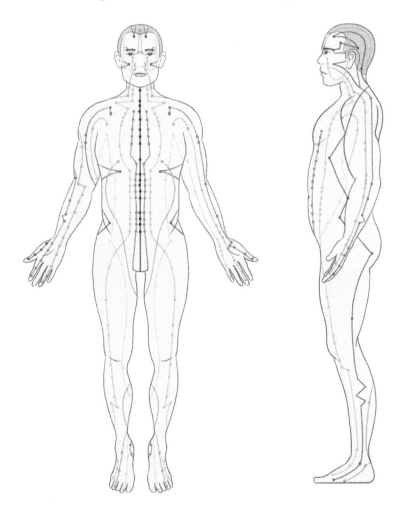

Each energy meridian is governed by yin and yang, the two types of energy. Yin and yang are continually flowing to achieve equilibrium in people, animals, and nature. The ancient art of qigong describes the two sides as two hands, where one is expressing and the other is recharging. This undoubtedly is why yin and yang are frequently alluded to when discussing relationships. Sometimes in a relationship, you must express the love and let the other be fed by it. Other times, it will be your turn to receive the nurturing. This is also where the idea that one can't pour from an empty cup was taken from. Energy is passed back and forth in all relationships.

Yin represents the feminine side of nature, encompassing darkness, tranquility, expansion, depth, cold, wetness, the moon, and water. Yang represents the masculine, encompassing light, activity, height, contraction, heat, dryness, heaven, the sun, and fire. Traditionally yin and yang are represented by a circle. These two pairs are constantly fluctuating to achieve balance. Yin flows up and yang flows down and must be balanced to achieve harmony within the body.

Acupressure is the art of pressing on a meridian point to encourage qi flow along that meridian. By relieving blockages, life energy can flow freely throughout the body to heal itself.

Beautiful Breathing

Respiration is essential for muscles to relax and let go. In Native American medicine, the connecting breath between beings happens when two people connect their touch during a quick gaspy breath.

A deep breath can activate the parasympathetic nervous system, which slows the heart rate and causes the body to relax and the mind to slow down as well. Breathing in deeply and holding the breath increases intra-abdominal pressure, thereby stimulating the vagus nerve (a major parasympathetic nerve). This sends signals to the brain and the body that reduce the fight-or-flight part of the autonomic nervous system (sympathetic nervous system).

Even something as simple as controlling the breath can have a profound impact on reducing emotional pain, especially if there has been tension in the relationship. Try some of these breathing exercises with your partner:

BOXED BREATHING: Breathe in for a count of 4, hold for a count of 4, and breathe out for a count of 4. Repeat this process 3 to 5 times.

4-7-8 BREATHING: Breathe in for a count of 4, hold the breath for a count of 7, and breathe out for a count of 8.

STIMULATING BREATHING: Breathe in and out of your nose as quickly as possible, trying for 3 cycles per second for no more than 15 seconds on your first try.

ZEN BREATH COUNTING: Exhale for a count of 1, then inhale for a count of 2, exhale for 2, then inhale for 3 and exhale for 3, and so on.

PURSED LIP BREATHING: Purse your lips and breathe out twice as long as you breathe in.

DIAPHRAGMATIC BREATHING: Put your hands on your belly so you can feel expansion in your diaphragm (the muscle that helps you breathe). Breathe in for a count of 4, and breathe out for a count of 8. Repeat 3 times.

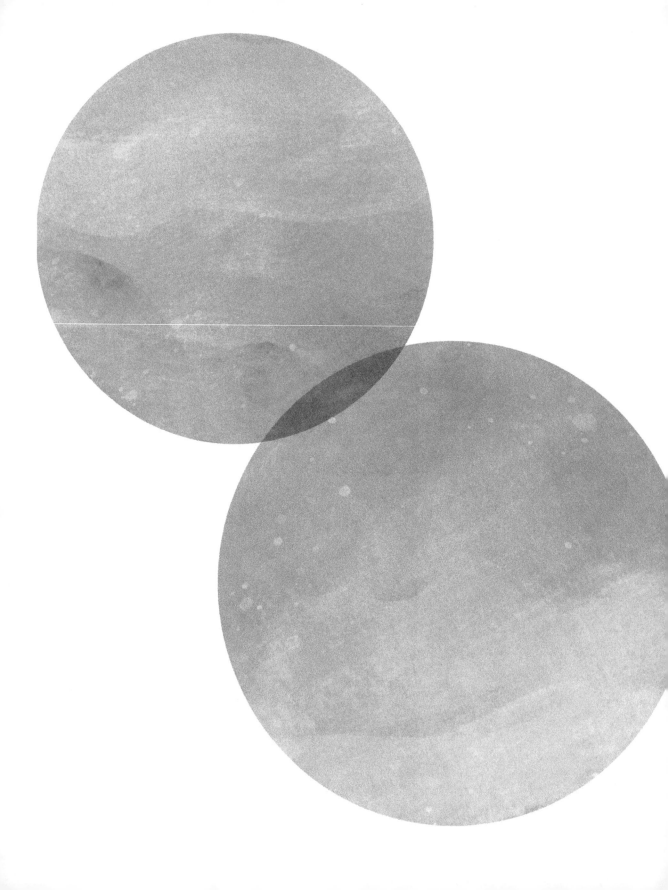

Chapter 2

For Love and Intimacy

The art and mastery of touch is a valuable tool in building, maintaining, and rekindling a strong relationship. It can help you better understand and meet the love language that your significant other speaks, as well as recognize and clarify your very own. Everyone desires to have their needs met in order for growth and fulfillment to occur. Engaging in an activity of dual immersion that requires give-and-take can help you relate to each other, and strengthen your mind-body connection to be able to understand your own actions and motives in a better light. By creating balance in the relationship, massage therapy can boost communication, helping you communicate both verbally and physically in a more efficient manner. It can be as simple or as complex as you choose to make it to create more balance and healthy intimacy in your relationship. The best part is, it's not expensive. You can simply use the tools that are already at your fingertips and start growing with your partner right now.

Love Languages
and Erotic Intelligence

In chapter 1 we spoke about the hormone changes that occur during a massage. Many of these changes involve neurohormones, which affect the nervous system and brain chemistry. These chemicals include dopamine, serotonin, epinephrine, and oxytocin.

Dopamine is a pleasure chemical in the body. During a massage, levels of dopamine increase. Dopamine is primarily associated with reward-related activities. The anticipation of the reward elevates the dopamine level in the cells. It influences fine motor activities like drawing, painting, or playing an instrument. It affects intuition, inspiration, joy, and enthusiasm. Without dopamine, we exhibit clumsiness and poor focus and can be easily distracted.

Serotonin, increased during massage, regulates emotional behavior, mood, social behavior, appetite, digestion, sleep, memory, sexual desire, and sexual function. It can cause irritability or cravings for sex or food. Those low in serotonin often tend to suffer from depression and obsessive-compulsive disorders. Serotonin is often referred to as the "happy" chemical in the brain because of its link to happiness and well-being.

Epinephrine or adrenaline levels are released during massage by stimulating the sympathetic nervous system. A quick invigorating massage can increase a person's alertness. Massage has been proven to reduce levels of cortisol, the stress-related neurohormone produced by the adrenal glands, which also produce epinephrine.

Touch is often associated with the release of oxytocin. It is sometimes referred to as the "love hormone," because of its relation to hugging, massage, and even orgasm. It has been proven to help with signs of anxiety, depression, and intestinal problems. It is heavily related to social bonding and sexual reproduction. It's most often connected with feelings of attachment during pregnancy, birthing, and lactation. Massage can strengthen your bond with your partner due to the release of hormones that are related to bonding and happiness.

Massage can help strengthen erotic intelligence between partners. Erotic intelligence is all about the capacity to trust yourself and be in touch with your own self, your body, your values, and your energy. To strengthen our mind-body connection we need to unblock patterns in our body and even in our relationships. Adding massage to your routine can help with building erotic intelligence and strengthening relationships.

Sharing Desires and Intentions

One of the most often overlooked steps of giving a good massage is setting the intention for the massage. In the treatment room, I will ask my clients what brought them in that day, what they want to focus on, what kind of pressure they like, and how I can help them. This helps me set my intention for the massage. If I miss their reason for coming in, they may be unhappy, or I may not be able to fulfill their needs for coming into the office for massage.

At home with your significant other, you can start by asking how your partner's day was. Do they have any aches or pains? Did sitting at their desk cause their neck or lower back to hurt? Did they have a tense meeting and wear their shoulders as earrings? Did they go to the gym and work a specific body part today? Communicating with your partner about their day is one of the best ways to learn how the massage might benefit them.

Other ways the massage will benefit a couple may be found through identifying each partner's love language and incorporating it into the massage. Someone whose strength is words of affirmation may desire to hear how well they are doing or be alerted when their partner hits a bothersome spot just right. A person who enjoys giving gifts may enjoy presenting the massage as one, perhaps as a coupon for massage to be playfully redeemed. Massage is an enjoyable activity for those who desire giving and receiving acts of service, because massage cannot be done solitarily. Massage is appealing to those who desire physical touch because it requires using your hands to manipulate tissues of the body. The options are endless when you know and cater to your partner's needs.

This is also a great time to ask about their feelings regarding massage or what kind of pressure they like. In the event that your significant other doesn't have a specific pain they wish to alleviate, consider setting an intention that involves relaxing together, getting to know each other's bodies, meeting each other's love languages, or even just spending time together.

Setting the Stage

A massage can be given anywhere that you are comfortable. My former husband and I often enjoyed nice quiet evenings massaging each other's feet on the couch. I have a friend whose husband has an entire room complete with a massage table set up just for her. A former boyfriend made a blanket fort in the middle of his living room and lit a ton of candles before very sweetly trying to rub my back. Your massage space can be elaborate or simple. It can be a couch, a bed, an ottoman, a chair, or even the floor—whatever feels comfortable to both of you. For added comfort, you may wish to place a pillow under the head and behind the knees of the massage recipient if lying on the back, or under the head and ankles if lying facedown. Always make sure your significant other is warm enough by adjusting the temperature in the room or covering them with a blanket. If you are worried about getting oil or lotion on the surface you are working on, I would also suggest covering the area with an extra sheet, blanket, or towel. Comfort is key when it comes to location.

Essential oils, lighting, and music are all great ways to change the mood, especially after a long day. The olfactory system, which detects smell, is part of the limbic system, which is related to emotions and learning, making it a really great way to increase time bonding through massage. Aromatherapy is a versatile way to enhance the massage experience. A variety of oils can add to the therapeutic element of the session, encouraging effects of relaxation, energy, or even sleep. The oils may be added to a diffuser based on the intentions set for the session. They may also be added to the lotion for quicker transdermal absorption. You can add essential oils to your massage oil or lotion as well. I personally prefer oil for home use, such as coconut, grape-seed, almond, corn, or even olive oil. Most store-bought lotions have a sticking feeling, require you to use a ton, and can leave you with an overwhelming aroma. I much prefer to use a simple oil and microwave it.

When adding an essential oil to a carrier oil (a fat-based substance used to disperse an essential oil), use 6 to 12 drops per ounce of lotion or oil. Certain oils such as cinnamon, ginger, spearmint, wintergreen, or peppermint will require less to prevent burning. Be aware that citrus oils (lemon, orange, lime, bergamot, grapefruit) increase the skin's sensitivity to light and may be better diffused. Make sure to ask your partner if they have any allergies before applying oils. If they have a nut allergy, be sure to avoid oils containing nuts. Review the section titled Oils, Lotions, and Sexy Love Potions in chapter 4 (page 48) for more suggestions on this.

If you wish to microwave a wet towel for 30 seconds to a minute and add essential oils, it can also enhance the relaxing experience. Just remember: If the towel is too warm when you press it to your forearm, it's going to be too warm for your partner. Apply it to the back or neck to warm up the tissue before a massage. The towel will remain warm for 1 to 2 minutes; after that you will want to remove it from their skin because it will be cold. Essential oils can also be added to a foot basin or warm bath after the massage for further enjoyment.

Incense and candles are another great way to appeal to the senses during a massage. One of our local holistic shops has an incense for anything your heart may desire. Lighting a few candles can help set the tone for your massage, as well. Make sure your choice of candle is not a mood killer or won't induce a headache if your partner is sensitive to smells. One of my favorite candles to buy for home use is the lotion candle. The wax around the wick melts into a warm massage lotion. It's a lot of fun to have a warm lubricant and it smells great.

Don't forget the music! Music is just as important for setting the mood as candles and a place to massage. Nothing ruins a massage quicker than a quick tempo or cheesy lyrics. If your partner has been through any trauma, then make sure you avoid music with tones, sound effects, or anything that may trigger them to become uncomfortable. Some people enjoy instrumentals of popular music; others can't stop their mind from singing the lyrics that aren't there. Ask your partner about music preference. There are many premade playlists and stations readily available. I would recommend a subscription to avoid the discomfort of a commercial interruption in the middle of the massage.

Giving and Receiving

Giving a massage can be just as much fun as getting a massage. It can be a great way to show your significant other that you care, carry out each of your love languages, or even help them eliminate an everyday ache or pain. Suppose your partner is complaining about how bad their feet hurt or that their neck has been bothering them. To me that sounds like the perfect opportunity to suggest a massage. They are practically asking you to massage them. Maybe your significant other is having a rough workweek or has finally reached a tough deadline. It may be the very reason for a foot massage and ice cream on the couch. Extend the invitation and see how they feel. You could also schedule a time for the end of the workweek so your partner can look forward to a relaxing massage ahead. One day you will need the same and if you act in kindness and show your regard for them, they will return the favor when they feel up for it.

Discussing any insecurities or worries about giving and receiving massage in a relationship can be helpful when adding this element to your relationship. Plan to stay engaged and check in with your partner about pressure or sensitive areas. Are they worried about what you will think about their body? Work like a trained massage therapist and keep all areas draped, only undraping the area as you go and re-covering it when it's done, or under dimmer lighting. Did they grow up in a home void of touch? That's understandable, and starting small and fully clothed may be a great option. It's also a good idea to ask what they like and don't like. This will make the massage more relaxing for both of you.

Remember that a massage doesn't have to be perfect to be a relaxing and worthwhile experience. You just have to make an effort. Any nervous energy may be correlated to an energy imbalance within the relationship. Effort helps balance the masculine and feminine energies in the relationship. When energies run high or dry and the qi of the relationship becomes off-kilter, quiet time engaged in massage can help. Even the professionals that win the world championship of massage started somewhere, and more than likely it was just like you—at home, practicing with someone they loved.

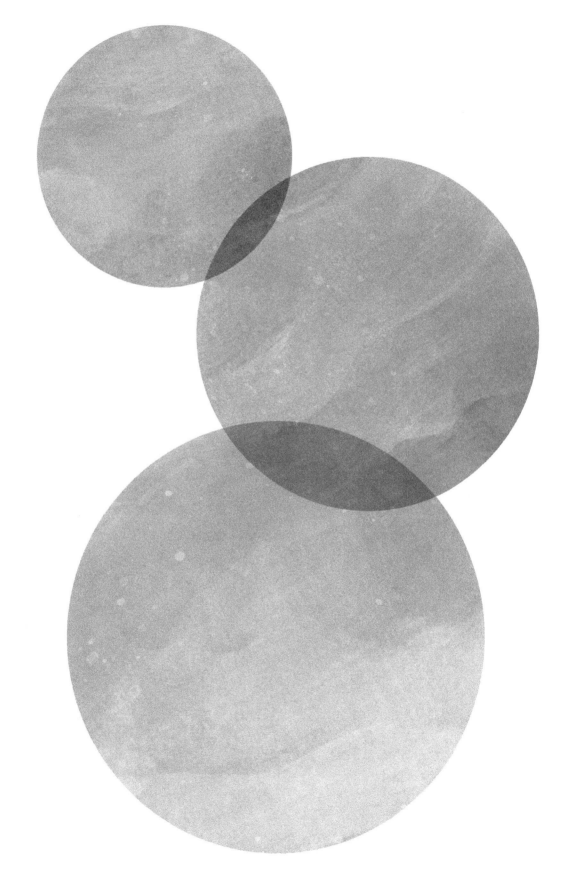

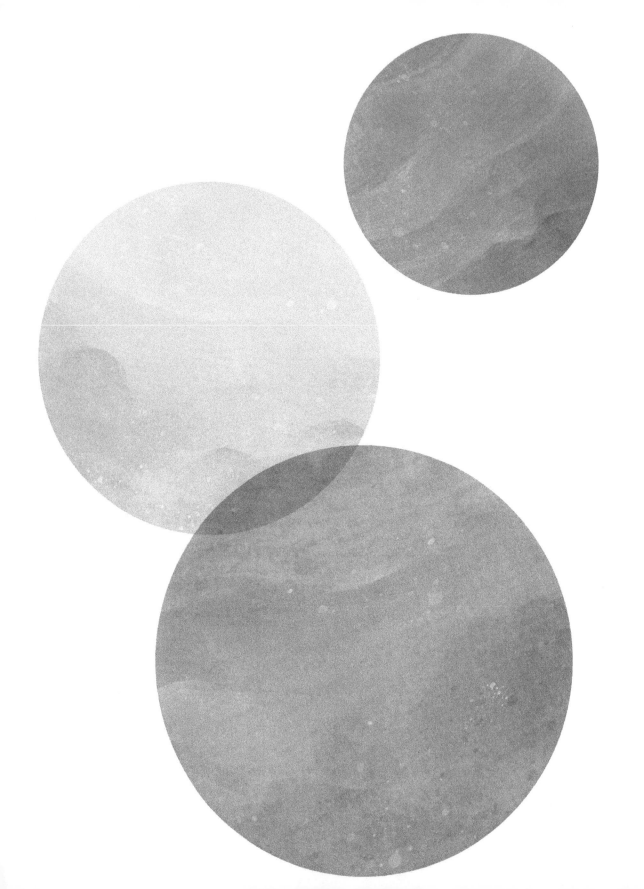

Part 2

BUILD YOUR SKILLS

Your new massage abilities start here. In this part of the book, we'll explore the wisdom in your hands, your feelings as you massage your partner, and how you can identify areas of tension and discomfort with your hands. You'll learn about the different physical sources of constriction, including adhesions and knots. Then you'll learn the simple stroke techniques that massage therapists have used and refined for decades—or perhaps centuries. Each technique offers unique benefits, soothing and relaxing muscles in various ways so that you can customize each massage. I encourage you to practice these techniques on your partner, using different levels of pressure and discussing with them which styles of touch they enjoy on which areas of their body. This part of the book will help you understand your partner, their body, and your capacity to offer healing and inspiring touch. Enjoy.

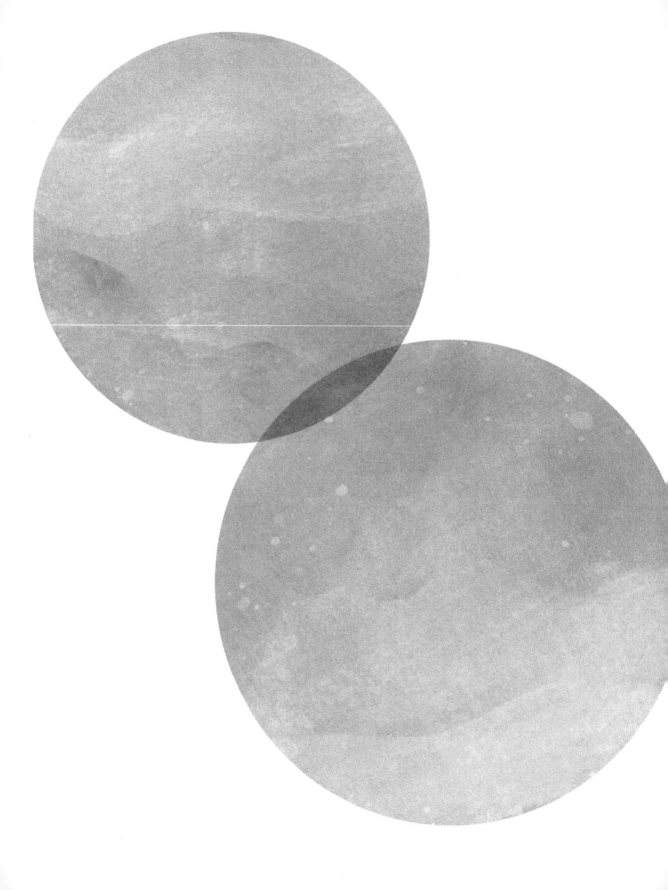

Chapter 3

The Wisdom in Your Hands

One of my favorite things is when clients tell me that their partner found a little knot or adhesion under their skin and tried to massage it out for them. Perhaps they got some relief, but typically they feel there's more work to do so they've come to my office. It's a very sweet act of love between partners. Oftentimes, they know it helped make them feel a little better, but their partners' hands got tired or it caused pain elsewhere. They've already realized the healing power of massage on their own.

Part of building your relationship with touch is learning how to respond to your partner and refine the sensitivity in your hands. By the time we are done you will feel confident about your massage skills and be able to use soothing touch as another tool for building a happy, healthy relationship. In this section, we'll discuss different styles of massage to help your partner relax as well as to aid in specific aches and pains. We will discuss classic strokes and age-old techniques from all over the world to enhance your massage skills.

Overview of Styles of Touch

We all have different tolerance levels for pressure and styles of massage. A firmer, deeper pressure may cause someone to fear being injured or hurt, whereas a nurturing touch may annoy the tense individual needing the heavy pressure. The best way to know what kind of pressure to use is to continuously check in with the receiver when you are giving the massage. Here are some good questions to ask your partner:

- Are you comfortable?

- Are you warm enough?

- Would you like more pressure?

- Would you like less pressure?

One of the keys to a good massage is an open line of communication, where you feel comfortable giving constructive criticism and taking that feedback and applying it to the massage. If your partner is weary of telling you, for whatever reason, watch for signs of agitation. These may include tensing up, twitching, or drawing away from you or even pained facial expressions. Adjust your pressure accordingly. You do not want to cause your partner pain or injury of any kind. If you are having an argument or disagreement prior to the massage, it may be best to first clear the air before giving or receiving a massage. This should be a time when you both feel safe. When conflict is brought into the massage session, it may disrupt the good feelings that come with giving and receiving a massage.

If an area is too sensitive or if the area is guarded due to emotions or former injuries, then use a lighter pressure or avoid it entirely. To decrease the pressure, you want to reduce the surface area of the body part and apply the pressure. If you were using a knee on the hamstrings and it was too much, then you might want to try a forearm, a fist, a flat hand, and lastly light fingertip pressure. Sometimes using a broader surface may be less painful in sensitive areas where fingertip pressure is too pokey and uncomfortable, but the broad fleshy part of the palm and fingers distributes the same amount of pressure more evenly and painlessly.

Using body parts other than the hands, such as the forearms, elbows, and even the shins, knees, and feet, may take excessive strain off the hands and wrists. The secret to being able to massage for long periods of time is good body mechanics. Instead of bending over your significant other, you may want to squat or lunge to prevent the force of gravity from wearing you down and causing you to tire early. Conserve your energy by avoiding heavy pressure over the joints, the lower back, ribs, back of the knee, front of the neck, and sternum. Areas of pressure over these areas have a potential to cause injury. In the event that you feel a pulse, always back off. Applying more pressure when you feel a pulse can impede blood flow and result in injury. Areas that require extra caution are called endangerment sites.

You don't have to avoid endangerment sites; they just require delicate touch to avoid damage. Always communicate this with your significant other. Sometimes that pain means there is an injury or it's time to visit a medical professional. Use your best judgment. A kind touch will build trust in your relationship; a painful touch will make your significant other afraid of your touch. Being confident in your ability to relieve your partner's pain can be fulfilling, and can strengthen your trust and dependence on one another.

Heavy pressure is great over large, broad areas of the body where there are larger, stronger muscles. Avoid heavy pressure over bony areas such as directly over the spine, floating ribs, and xiphoid process (the very bottom part of the sternum that lies between the ribs), which may be very uncomfortable. Nerves create sharp electrical pain. In the event that your partner alerts you of something that elicits a nerve response, adjust your technique to accommodate the area. Other areas, such as the large muscles of the back, glutes, hamstrings, and quads, are capable of taking a shocking amount of pressure. Smaller body areas just need less pressure.

Hand Strength

Many people worry that they need to have strong hands in order to give a great massage. The truth is, you don't have to use your hands all the time. You can alternate between using your fingers, knuckles, fists, forearms, elbows, and even a knee or your glutes to sit on the area. Having good body mechanics and not hunching over the area that you are working on will sustain you and allow you to work deeper and longer.

At home, you may be more inclined to do shorter massage sessions, so we won't need to focus on this as much. However, even for home massage, it's helpful to keep your hands slightly cupped and relaxed rather than locking your joints and pushing in with heavy pressure. Try to keep your wrists in a normal, relaxed position when using the forearm or elbows. When massaging larger muscle groups like the glutes or buttocks, you could use a fist, elbow, or knee instead of a thumb or fingers, because those stronger muscles can handle some more pressure.

If your hands become sore, use a tool such as a lacrosse or golf ball. Switch the position of your body, or try using a different part of your body to do the massage. Also check in with your partner to see how they feel about the sensation or pressure. Giving a massage should feel like a fairly natural activity for your body—not a workout. If you feel sore or tired after giving a massage, keep practicing and continue to use your hands and body in different ways.

Knots, Tension, and Messages from the Hands

I have often had to demystify the knot, adhesion, and trigger points for not only my clients, but members of the massage community as well. An adhesion is two surfaces that are stuck together, which restricts movement. A knot is a broader term referring to anything that can be felt under the skin. It can be a trigger point or an adhesion. It is more widely recognized as anything that affects movement. Basically, it's a disrupter in the body, stirring up chaos. It's creating imbalance and disrupting normal homeostasis. It's not specific. It's a pretty general, broad term for that thing that can be felt, but not 100 percent explained.

Fascia is present throughout the entire body and can run from head to toe. The fascial layer responds to heat and movement by melting and moving more easily. Fascia becomes thicker and harder around injuries due to dehydration, lack of circulation, or lack of movement. Because fascia is made up of collagen fibers, as scars are also made of collagen, sometimes people will refer to fascia as scar tissue.

Massage produces heat and movement. Methods of breaking up adhesions in the fascia traditionally involve fractioning and compressing a scar as many different ways as possible to break down the collagen fibers that have grown into the tissue. This is why some techniques are slower or faster in breaking up adhesions. They produce more circulation or heat than other methods. This may also be why Chinese medicine also claims that heat drives out heat, and explains why sometimes heat helps better than ice when applied to the body. Cold moves old blood out of an area so fresh oxygenated blood can move back in. Heat causes blood to pool to the area.

Because this adhesion is restricting movement, it may cause pain by pulling on different structures, such as nerves, other muscles, tendons, or ligaments. One of the main characteristics of muscles is that they are able to shorten and lengthen. This differentiates them from other body tissues. An adhesion keeps a muscle from reaching its full extensible length. To the hands, this area may feel thicker than the surrounding tissue. You may notice crackling or plastic-wrap-type noises from this area. Whenever you stretch an area, you may additionally notice a popping noise. Don't panic. These sounds don't mean you have injured your partner. Most of the time these sounds are what we call "spontaneous realignment."

Releasing the muscle may cause the skeletal system to realign. Muscles pull bones out of place. This may be a rib or vertebra sliding back into place, or trapped air being released. Because of these movements, metabolic waste trapped in the tissue is flushed out. This is why it is always suggested that you drink lots of water after a massage. The body is reabsorbing and processing the waste trapped in the cells and water is a great way to support this work.

Working with Trigger Points

Trigger points are contracted "sarcomere," small units of muscle cells within the muscle. These can affect the movement of the muscle. Trigger-point work is great, because it has the potential to soothe multiple areas of pain around the body all at once, since trigger points can cause referred pain, or pain in an area of the body other than where it originates. When contracted, they can cause pain and sensitivity to the touch or the surface, and may be so hard and tight that the recipient feels nothing due to the degree and length of time that they have been contracted.

If you were to glide your hands across the skin, you may feel a difference in suppleness. The tissue may be hard or even lumpy. If you were to attempt to pick the skin up off the muscle and roll it, you would notice an adhesed or stuck area that doesn't let go. It may even hurt, be tender, or pinch. Sometimes adhesions are compared to hard raisins under the skin. Most of the time when these muscle cells finally release or let go, they may do it in an abrupt way.

For example, there is a trigger point in the calf that refers to pain in the jaw. A trigger point in the neck may refer over the side of the head or behind the eye. These points may refer pain locally or even cause pain to travel to a different, unrelated area, which the nervous system is responsible for relaying. The theory of where the trigger points refer pain to is based on the work of Janet Travell, who found that different spots of tenderness and irritability referred to other areas, and began to chart them.

To release areas, you can try a couple of different techniques. You can gently mash the area with your fingers and try to compress the tissue until it releases, while instructing your partner to breathe. Sometimes this will cause a harder release within the muscle that almost makes it jerk. You can gently friction the area repeatedly by rubbing it over and over from different directions or in circles.

If your hands get tired, there's no shame in using a golf ball or lacrosse ball over the area gently. You can try to pick the skin up off the muscle and roll the area over it, pinching the areas that feel like bubble wrap. For some this may be a little too intense, so it is always better to work gently and carefully so that your partner doesn't bruise. The ultimate goal is to relieve pain, not to create more pain. After the massage, a nice warm bath with Epsom salts, an ice pack on the sore spot, or even a topical pain-relief cream may be a comforting touch to your partner.

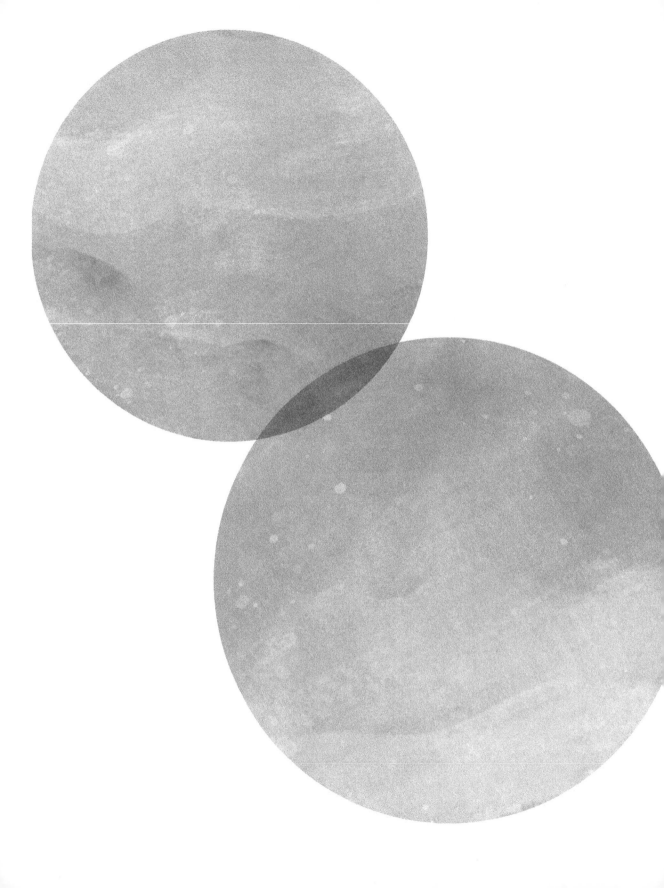

Chapter 4

Stroke Techniques

Some people love heavy pressure. Other people will jump off the table and run away if you use heavy pressure on them. Although some like a nice slow massage, others may find them annoying. They prefer a fast massage that gets the blood pumping. Some techniques may calm your mind and melt you like butter, maybe even putting you to sleep.

Communication and the spirit of adventure can liven up your relationship as well as potentially alter its physical and emotional aspects. Massage strokes or techniques for performing massage can have different effects on the physical composition of the body and the emotional aspect of the body. As we know, we are not only altering the fascia (the fibrous connective tissue layer under the skin) and adhesions under the skin, but also causing the body to release neurohormones. These neurohormones affect mood, attachment, and even bodily functions. Here are some basic traditional techniques that we will build on throughout this book to help you get started. Feel free to reference these terms and images at any point while working your way through this book with your partner, as a refresher.

Effleurage

Effleurage is a gliding Swedish massage stroke made with the palm of the hand. It is a gentle movement with broad pressure.

BENEFITS: Effleurage is a great technique to start a massage, because it is extremely effective for applying lubricants evenly to the skin. It is helpful for relaxing your partner and getting them accustomed to your touch as a first stroke. It is a great way to gauge comfort and pressure. It is the building block for establishing trust between the giver and the receiver. Effleurage will help you locate areas that may be adhesed or tender. This technique helps get blood flow to improve circulation and move lymph, which helps remove waste from the tissues.

CHARACTERISTICS: Soothing, relaxing, acclimating

1. Apply lotion or oil to your hands, and then run the flat hand up and down the body part in a gliding motion.

2. Check in with your partner about pressure. For more pressure, lean more into the stroke or use the knuckles of a closed fist. Be sure to keep your back straight and use your legs to push your body forward into the stroke. Always try to work toward the torso to help the flow of blood back toward the heart.

3. Use longer, slower strokes to soothe your significant other, or use shorter strokes for an area of pain or discomfort. This stroke is best when using two hands evenly over the body, mirroring each other or moving them in opposite directions at the same time. It may be done in a straight line, in wavelike motions, or even in circular motions.

4. To move on to another body part or end the massage, use a version of effleurage called feathering, or the nerve stroke, by slowly lightening up your pressure till you are using your fingertips only and continue to lighten the pressure over the area until you take your hands away.

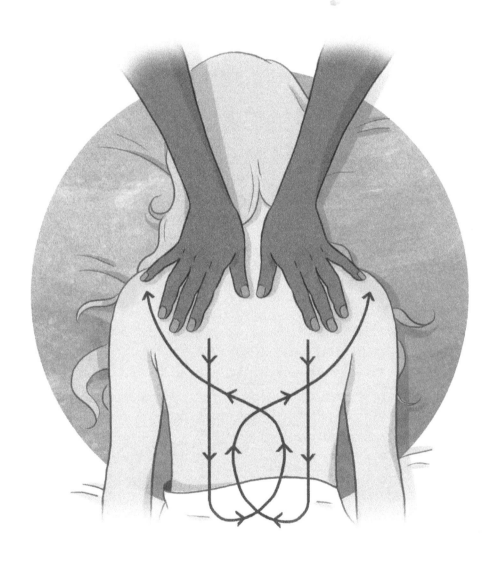

Petrissage (Kneading)

Petrissage comes from the French word "pétrir," which means "to knead." Petrissage is a Swedish massage stroke used to compress and lift underlying tissue. Other variations of petrissage may include kneading, wringing, and skin rolling. It is used for working deep into fleshy areas of the body in a rhythmic motion.

BENEFITS: Helps separate the layers of tissue from one another to release and remove adhesions. Increases circulation to the area. Breaks up areas of congestion. Loosens tissue layers. Distributes energy.

CHARACTERISTICS: Loosening, penetrating, separating

1. Petrissage is done most easily with tissue that has been warmed up using effleurage or friction. Begin by applying oil or lotion to the skin. Perform some effleurage, gliding your hands up around the area to help increase circulation.

2. Position your hands like you would grasp handlebars or as if they were even crab claws, by slightly cupping them but bringing the thumb slightly out to grasp the tissue. Graze the tissue with your fingertips while lifting it. You may do this single-handed or while alternating both hands.

3. In the event that your hands get tired, you may make two fists, and alternate them while twisting them into the tissue. Try to find a comfortable rhythm or tempo while repeating this motion.

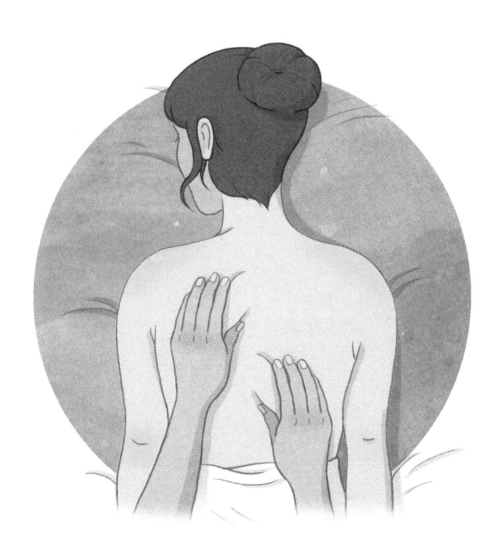

Circling (Circular Friction)

Circling can be done with the palms of the hands for a more effleurage-like technique, or with the fingertips, thumbs, fist, or heel of the hand to produce more of a friction-type effect that's more point-specific.

BENEFITS: Circling helps increase circulation through the vigorous movement of fluids. It can be used to disperse stagnant energy.

CHARACTERISTICS: Stimulating, invigorating

1. Apply oil or lotion to the surface you wish to massage.
2. Using the tips of your fingers or the palms of your hands, make figure-eight movements, working down both sides of the back at the same time. Alternatively, use your forearms, rotating them back and forth if your hands become tired.

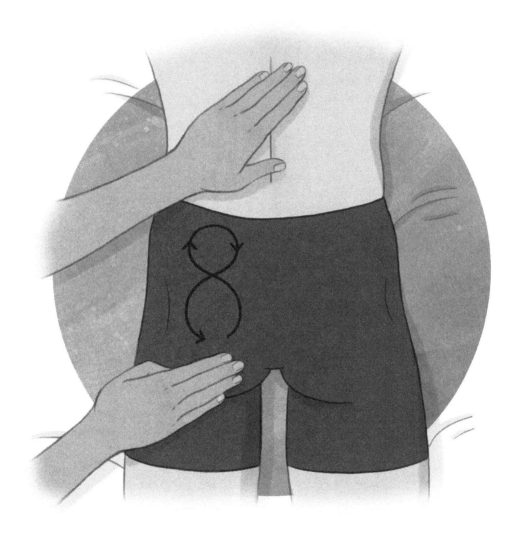

Compression

Compression is the act of applying steady pressure to an area and holding it. As the tissue layers relax and separate, you may feel as though you are moving even though you remain still.

BENEFITS: Compression improves the flow of circulation by forcing blood into a stiff area. It is an effective technique that can cause a lot of change when held. In Eastern techniques, it is used to gather energy to the area.

CHARACTERISTICS: Healing, energetic, pain-relieving, warming

1. Locate a knot, adhesion, or tight area in the musculature. Apply steady pressure to the area with your fingers, thumbs, palms, fist, forearm, elbow, or even your knee if it is a large broad area such as the hamstring or glutes. Hold the area for 15 to 20 seconds or until you feel the area release.

2. Move on to the next area.

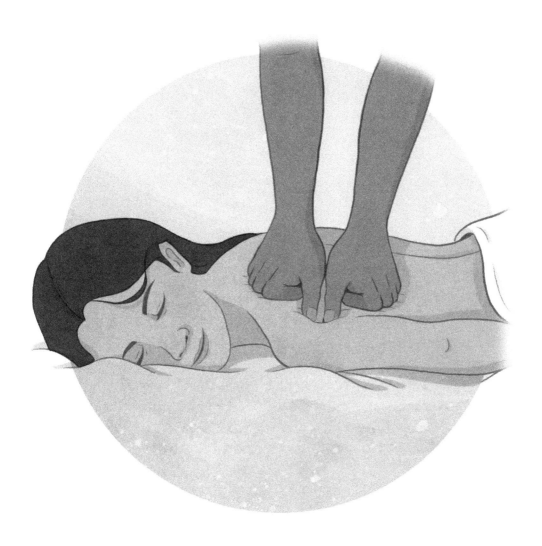

Friction

Friction is a technique that involves repeatedly making short back-and-forth motions with the thumbs, fingers, elbows, or fists.

BENEFITS: Friction is an awesome technique for breaking up areas of stagnant energy and congestion. It is best done repeatedly and quickly or very slowly with a good amount of pressure to tight and adhesed areas. It is a good technique for working around bony areas. It may be done with the tips of the fingers or thumbs. The idea is to increase blood flow and force the adhesed areas to separate. This is a good technique to pair with trigger-point work or acupressure.

CHARACTERISTICS: Stimulating, invigorating, releasing

1. Use effleurage or petrissage to locate areas of tightness or adhesion. Communicate with your partner to find out if any areas are tender, sensitive, or painful.

2. Find an area that may feel like a taut band or cord. It may even feel like a thick pad under the skin. Check in with your significant other. This may or may not be an area of pain or tenderness.

3. Apply pressure while moving over the area, or hold slow, steady pressure to the site of tightness. Push into it until the area releases while instructing your partner to breathe. Alternatively, you may use a light level of pressure and use more repetitions of motion across the area to get the same effect.

4. As you work, you will feel the area become looser. If your partner experiences any increased tenderness or sharp or increasing pain, reduce the pressure or switch techniques.

5. If your fingers or hands become sore or the joints become sore, you may wish to purchase a Chinese soup spoon and gently scrape the area instead. If the area you are scraping begins to get red or have a small red spot, becomes raw, or gets increasingly hot, then you may want to stop.

6. Flush the area out using a gliding effleurage movement, preferably toward the lymph nodes.

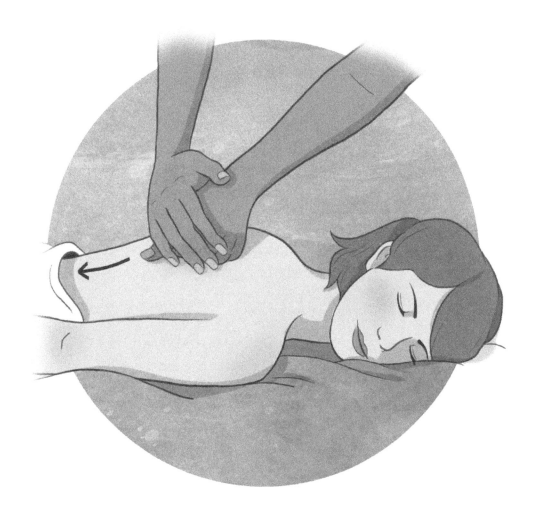

Stretching

Stretching involves taking the muscle to its longest length to free up structures under the skin.

BENEFITS: The act of stretching typically refers to taking a muscle that is shortened and lengthening it to increase blood flow. This in turn increases flexibility and range of motion.

CHARACTERISTICS: Energizing, invigorating, stimulating

1. Run your hands over the tight muscle of your partner to locate the joint it crosses.

2. Have your partner relax and move the joint through the movement that it performs while you move the part of the body farthest away from the torso. If you are working on the hip, shoulder, or fingers, you may move the body part in circles. If it is a finger joint, wrist, elbow, knee, or toe, then just move the joint in a bending motion as it would move normally.

3. Encourage the receiver to focus on breathing out more than in.

4. Every time you press into the stretch, hold the body part for a count of 20 to 30 seconds. You may also wish to observe your significant other's breathing and hold it while the chest rises 3 or 4 times. Check in with them regularly to make sure they are not in pain or distress. Never force the joint past what feels comfortable, as you do not want to dislocate or damage the joint.

5. You may repeat taking the joint through the range of motion up to 3 times. Be gentle. The last thing you want to do is be forceful and cause your receiver to tense up and injure you or them.

6. Return the body part to its normal position. A great way to transition from this stroke is to shake or rock the area, or move back into effleurage, pushing blood flow back toward the torso.

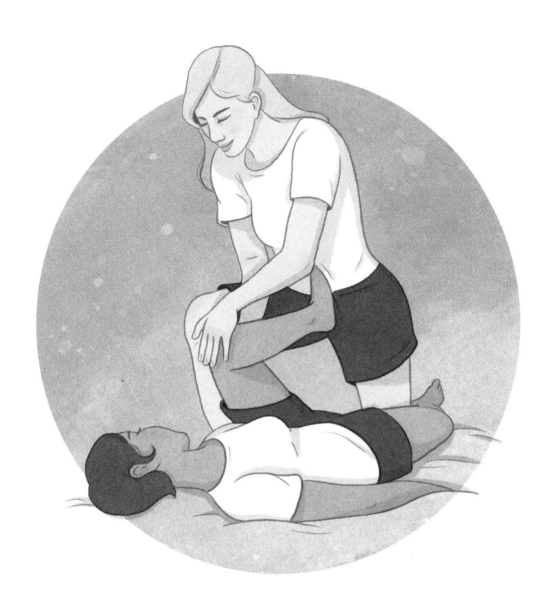

Percussion (Tapotement)

Although most massage techniques are relaxing, percussion is quite the opposite, promoting stimulating effects. It involves striking the body with alternating hands for therapeutic effects.

BENEFITS: Tapotement is a great way to break up congestion in the chest. It can help tone and slowly free up contracted muscles by slowly jarring them into relaxation. It's also a great way to free up stagnant energy.

CHARACTERISTICS: Stimulating, invigorating

1. Warm your partner's body with some light effleurage or compression to get the recipient used to your touch.

2. Next, use two cupped hands, the pinky side of a fist, or the pinky side of the blade of the hand (where palms point toward each other) to gently and rhythmically pound the tissue.

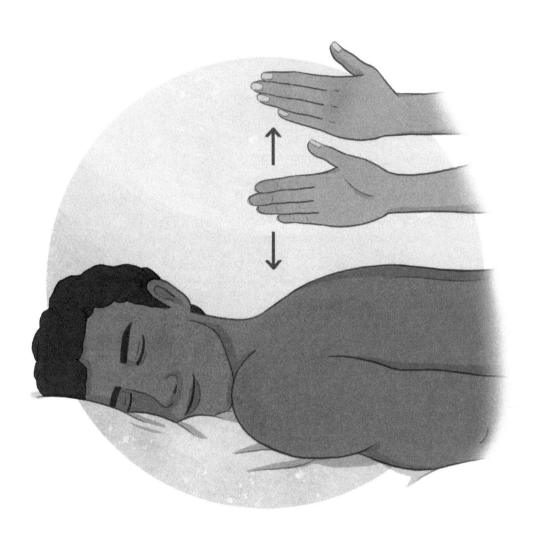

Oils, Lotions, and Sexy Love Potions

Essential oils can be a great way to add sensual therapeutic benefits to any massage. Recently I had the pleasure of helping develop the essential oil program for massage therapists with Simply Earth, a therapeutic-grade essential oil company based in Wisconsin that gives back 13 percent of their profits every month to an organization that fights human trafficking.

Essential oils are concentrated, plant-based oils that have a strong aroma. These therapeutic oils have many benefits for the mind and body, forming the healing modality known as aromatherapy. Oils are traditionally used by inhalation. Essential oils applied to the skin are absorbed into the bloodstream, delivering a range of benefits to the body systems and organs. Just inhaling the aroma of an essential oil can trigger memories and even various emotions, while influencing mood, hormones, and the nervous system.

A pure essential oil should never be applied directly to the skin, as it has the potential to cause skin damage when undiluted. Instead it should be diluted with a carrier oil at a dilution of typically no more than 2 percent, depending on the oil. This is typically 6 to 12 drops of essential oil per ounce of carrier oil. Some oils such as cinnamon, ginger, wintergreen, spearmint, and peppermint should be diluted even further due to the ability to burn or thin the blood. Always check for contraindications when combining essential oils with medications. In the event of a reaction, douse the area with carrier oil and repeatedly blot with a towel. Don't use water—it can increase irritation by spreading the oil.

Citrus oils tend to cause photosensitivity, so it's best to diffuse them. For 72 hours after application, one wouldn't want to get into a tanning bed, work out in the sun, or lie by the pool. If you have children at home, check the recommended age before application since their immune systems are still developing and they may have undiscovered allergies. If you are pregnant or breastfeeding, always check with your doctor before using essential oils.

Some of my favorite carrier oils are very easy to find both online and at your local grocery store:

FRACTIONATED COCONUT OIL is great for normal to dry skin types. It is thought to have anti-inflammatory properties, keep the skin moisturized, form a protective skin barrier, and help heal wounds, since it has medium-chain fatty acids due to antimicrobial properties that can help with acne and protect the skin from harmful bacteria.

GRAPE-SEED OIL is noncomedogenic and lightweight, making it good for all skin types. It has high levels of linoleic acid, which can help fight clogged pores, making it quite popular for use among massage therapists. Grape-seed oil is also a very good carrier oil to use for facials or for a moisturizer.

ALMOND OIL is good for dry skin, especially in the presence of eczema, psoriasis, or acne. This oil is thought to be helpful with rejuvenating cell turnover. Almond oil is also rich in vitamin E and vitamin K, making it a great choice for fine lines, wrinkles, and sun damage.

JOJOBA OIL is good for all skin types and is also known to help balance oily skin and help manage breakouts. This carrier oil is nongreasy and is also very moisturizing, making it great for massage.

Here are some recommended essential oil blends to help with everything from anxiety to lethargy.

CALMING ESSENTIAL OILS include lavender, jasmine, basil, bergamot, German chamomile, rose, ho wood, ylang ylang, frankincense, sandalwood, clary sage, patchouli, geranium, jasmine, marjoram, vetiver, rosemary, melissa, and neroli.

Recommended blends (all blended with a 4-ounce bottle of massage oil):

- 12 drops of lavender, 12 drops of sweet orange, 12 drops of bergamot, and 12 drops of ylang ylang

- 16 drops of lavender, 16 drops of lime, and 16 drops of spearmint

- 16 drops of lemon, 16 drops of lavender, and 16 drops of rosemary

- 16 drops of vetiver, 16 drops of patchouli, 8 drops of jasmine, and 8 drops of ho wood

INVIGORATING ESSENTIAL OILS include sweet orange, bergamot, lime, grapefruit, lemon, eucalyptus, basil, juniper berry, rosemary, peppermint, frankincense, spearmint, lavender, and sandalwood.

Recommended blends (all blended with a 4-ounce bottle of massage oil):

- 16 drops of juniper berry, 16 drops of orange, and 16 drops of grapefruit

- 24 drops of lemon and 24 drops of peppermint

- 16 drops of eucalyptus, 16 drops of peppermint, and 16 drops of rosemary

- 16 drops of lime, 16 drops of lemon, and 16 drops of grapefruit

CHEERFULNESS ESSENTIAL OILS are thought to help with improving one's mood and include chamomile, sweet orange, lavender, ginger, tangerine, frankincense, coriander, basil, clary sage, marjoram, lemon, orange, blood orange, lime, grapefruit, peppermint, ylang ylang, vetiver, grapefruit, bergamot, jasmine, and rose.

Recommended blends:

- 12 drops of bergamot, 12 drops of grapefruit, 12 drops of lemon, and 12 drops of lime

- 12 drops of lavender, 6 drops of jasmine, 6 drops of frankincense, and 12 drops of vetiver

- 12 drops of bergamot, 12 drops of tangerine, 12 drops of blood orange, and 12 drops of marjoram

- 16 drops of peppermint, 16 drops of lemon, and 16 drops of blood orange

AROUSING ESSENTIAL OILS include clary sage, lavender, sandalwood, ylang ylang, vanilla, Peru balsam, palmarosa, damiana, black pepper, neroli, rose, benzoin (similar to vanilla), Amyris, cinnamon, ginger, peppermint, jasmine, geranium, fennel, and patchouli.

Recommended blends:

- 16 drops of lavender, 6 drops of jasmine, 18 drops of Amyris, and 16 drops of peppermint

- 16 drops of ylang ylang, 16 drops of palmarosa, and 16 drops of patchouli

- 12 drops of sandalwood, 12 drops of ylang ylang, 12 drops of lavender, and 12 drops of neroli

- 16 drops of clary sage, 16 drops of juniper berry, and 16 drops of geranium

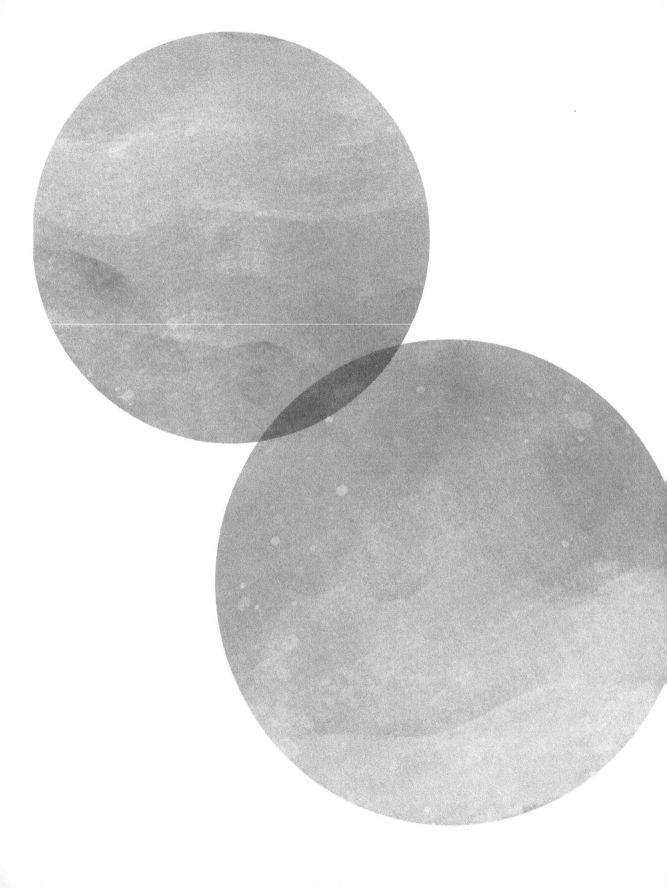

Chapter 5

Traditions and Methods

Much of Western massage practice aims to soothe the muscles and support the detoxification of tissues by increasing circulation and mobilizing the lymphatic system. It focuses on the physical anatomy as an arrangement of organs and systems. Eastern medicine, which dates back thousands of years, views the body as an integrated system of energies that are highly connected to our mind and emotions.

Most Eastern styles of massage rely on intuition and observations over time. Some focus on moving energy in the body through a network known as meridians. In this chapter, we will explore massage methods from different traditions in order to explore different ways to heal the mind, body, and spirit—and encourage a healthy and rewarding relationship with your partner. We will discuss each method of touch, its origin, and its specific healing properties, and give step-by-step instructions for performing them in the safety of your home with the one you love.

Shiatsu

Shiatsu is a Japanese word meaning "finger pressure." It uses "ki" instead of the Chinese "chi" to describe energy. Energy is more commonly synonymous with breath in both languages. Lots of attention is paid to the "hara," or abdomen, which rises and falls with breath. It uses the five elements to harmonize yin and yang and is similar to the Chinese "tui na." Shiatsu is also very similar to Thai massage, which has origins in Ayurvedic and Chinese medicine, because they are both done fully clothed on the floor on a mat and work energy lines. Shiatsu uses static, steady pressure of the foot, thumb, or palm on the energy lines, focusing deep firm pressure on them. That rhythmically used pressure pays special attention to relaxing joints and stretching muscles, and even stretching the meridian lines.

BASIC SHIATSU ROUTINE

1. Start your partner out lying facedown. Kneel beside them. Rub your hands together for 30 to 40 seconds while taking some deep breaths.

2. Make initial contact with your partner with the palms of your hands. Pay attention to the rhythm of your partner's breathing. Spend a few moments gently compressing your partner's back with an open palm.

3. Cross your arms to stretch the lower back, pressing into the lower back and the upper back. Hold for a few seconds.

4. Position your body into a lunging position on one knee. Apply pressure with your hands on either side, pointing away from the spine, straight down, keeping your joints aligned or "stacked." Move to the glute. Use an elbow to apply pressure to the glute. Walk your palms down the legs.

5. Bend the knee while pressing a flat palm into the glute or lower back so as not to raise it. Put both hands on the sacrum (the bone connecting the spine between the hips) and push in. Repeat on the other side of the body.

6. Next, kneel at the head. Press into the shoulders with your palms. Walk down both sides of the back with your palms; with stacked joints, apply perpendicular pressure.

7. Next, use your thumbs to friction the tissue on both sides of the spine all the way down. Return to the shoulders and use your thumbs to friction across the top of the shoulders.

8. Instruct your partner to roll over. Remain kneeling. Place your hands gently on their abdomen and observe their breath. Pick up their arm and move it to a 90-degree angle. Walk up and down the arm with flattened palms compressing the arm. Work your partner's palm by compressing the fingers gently and then pulling them.

9. Walk your palms down one leg. Then go to the other leg and walk your palms down that leg. Squat down and pick up your partner's feet. Rest your elbows on your thighs to stretch the spine. Swing the legs back and forth a few times from left to right. Lower the legs. Return to the shoulders and neck and compress them before trading places to receive.

PALMING

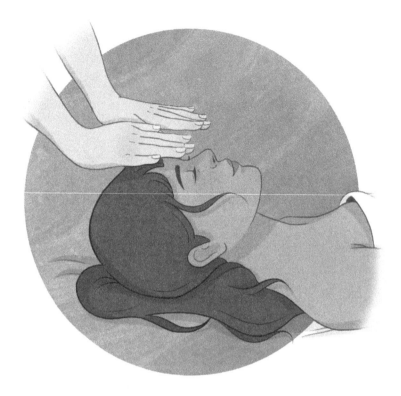

Palming is a form of compression with a flat palm, done on the floor.

1. Position your partner on the floor. Lunge or kneel, placing your flat palm into the area you are treating.

2. Hold pressure with your joints stacked over one another and your hand pushing straight down. Walk your flat palms down the meridian lines, holding as needed.

NECK STRETCH

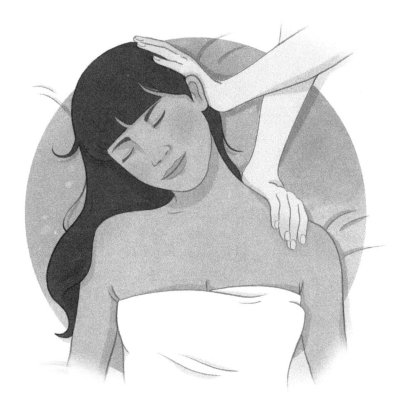

1. Start with your hands on both shoulders and the head straight. Reach one arm to the opposite side of the body. Use this arm to push the head gently toward the opposite shoulder. Hold this stretch for 10 to 15 seconds.

2. Move the head back to the midline of the body, and repeat on the opposite side.

SHOULDER COMPRESSIONS

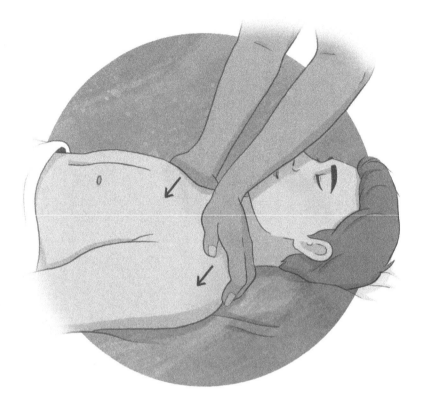

1. Position your partner faceup. Palm your hands across the chest, pulling the receiver gently into the mat and holding for 10 to 15 seconds to stretch the chest and pecs.

2. Next, move your hands to the tops of the shoulders below the earlobes. Turn the palms out. Push into the shoulders and hold for 10 to 15 seconds.

3. Alternating your hands, push into the shoulders for a few seconds apiece.

LEG STRETCH

1. Squat down and pick up your partner's feet. Rest your elbows on your thighs to stretch the spine.

2. Swing the legs back and forth a few times from left to right. Lower the legs.

Swedish

Swedish massage is based on the work of Peter Ling and was originally used to enhance athletic performance, much like our sports massage today. It primarily uses the following techniques for a relaxing massage experience. The massage is typically very fluid and connecting, utilizing long gliding strokes with light to firm pressure. It is the most popular type of massage.

WRINGING

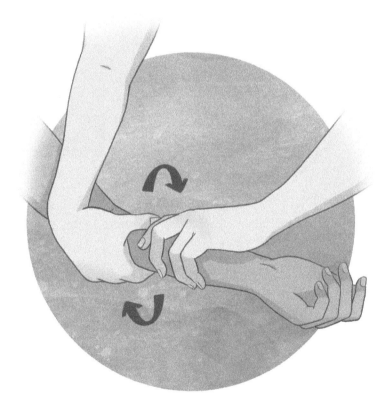

This technique is great for limbs.

1. Put one hand above the other hand, with the fingers facing in opposite directions.

2. Push your hands around the area, wrapping them around the limb. Move in circular movements back and forward, working up and down the body part.

SPREADING

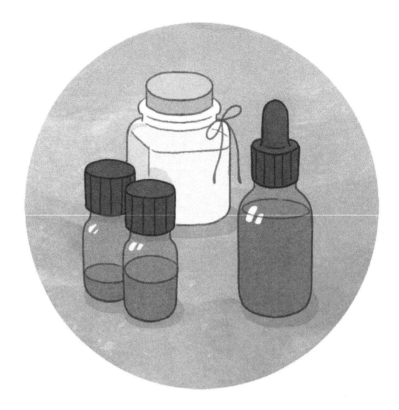

This technique helps open up the muscles and is great for the legs and arms.

1. Position your hands on both sides of the body part.

2. Compress and effleurage the area in a V-like shape, spreading the tissue and opening up the muscle to create blood flow. Do this rhythmically a few times, or do it and hold for 10 to 15 seconds.

VIBRATION

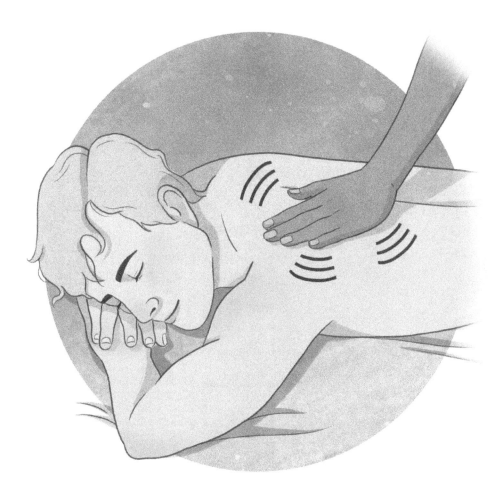

Vibration uses quick movements to loosen and warm up tissue.

1. Find the area you want to loosen or warm up.

2. Place a flat palm on the surface. Rub your hand back and forth quickly over the area.

SKIN ROLLING

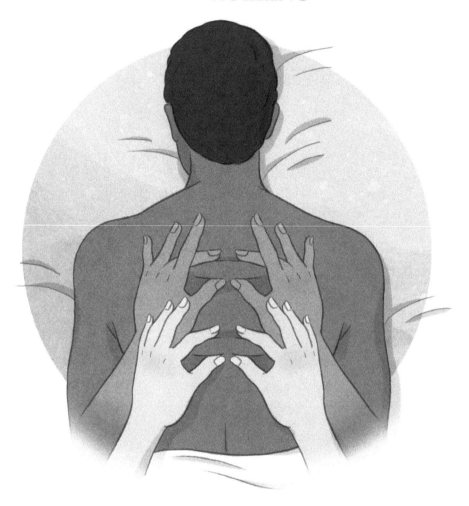

1. Warm up the tissue using effleurage.

2. Using the tips of your fingers, pick up the skin, lifting it off the muscle and bone. Walk your fingers down the area, keeping the tissue lifted up off the area as you go.

ROCKING OR JOSTLING

This is a great way to help relax the nervous system, especially when holding tension that causes us to stiffen up.

1. Place two hands about shoulder-width apart on an area.

2. Gently push the area back and forth to allow the movement to travel and loosen other areas.

CIRCUMDUCTION

This technique is often used with the fingers and toes.

1. Grasp the finger or toe and pull outward. Make tiny circular movements with the body part in its joint.

2. Reverse and move in the opposite direction before going on to the next finger or toe.

FEATHERING

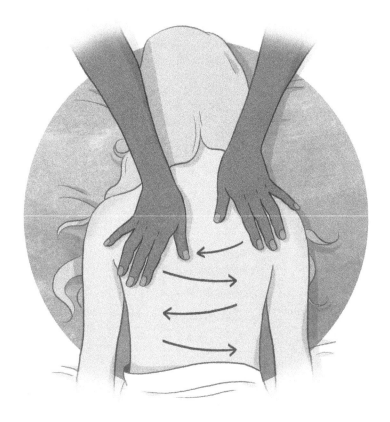

This technique is a great way to end working on one body part and transition to another.

1.   Lightly brush the skin with your fingertips. Alternate hands while keeping them relaxed.

2.   Make the pressure lighter and lighter until you come to a stopping point.

RAKING

1.   Spread the fingers apart and hook your fingertips into the tissue.

2.   Pull the hands back, alternating them while raking the hands across the back.

Deep Tissue

Deep tissue massage focuses on using heavier pressure combined with Swedish massage for more therapeutic benefits. The purpose of this massage is to realign deeper levels of tissue. The same principles are applied as to Swedish massage; however, the work is deeper and may focus on relieving more areas of stress and pain. Compressions are typically held longer to release trigger points and affect muscle tissue. Friction is very effective in the release of trigger points. Most of the time, it is followed by stretching or traction to realign the muscle fibers to prevent them from returning to their previous state.

Contrary to popular belief, this technique does not have to involve pain. The gentler use of massage techniques with more repetition can still have the same result; however, it may take more time to resolve. It may take up to one session per month that an issue has been occurring, so if an issue doesn't resolve, don't feel discouraged. In the event of nerve involvement, I always recommend seeing a professional for advanced techniques and to avoid inflaming the nerve. They may utilize the Swedish massage routine (page 59), while incorporating a few more point-specific techniques.

COMPRESS, HOLD, BREATHE

One of my favorite techniques that requires minimum effort is a myofascial technique.

1. Apply lotion to your forearm. Using your forearm, apply pressure straight down onto the area. Check with your partner to find out if the pressure is acceptable. Hold the compression and apply pressure until the fascia or muscle moves your arm itself.

2. Instruct your receiver to take long, slow, deep breaths. See the Beautiful Breathing sidebar (page 13) for breathing techniques.

3. Adjust your body weight to keep your joints stacked as your partner's muscles begin to relax themselves.

THE EDGE TECHNIQUE

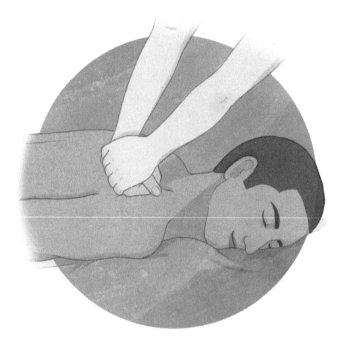

The purpose of this technique is to release trigger points or adhesions that lie deep in the tissue. Adjust your position right, left, up, or down if you feel a pulse while performing this technique, as it can impede blood flow.

1. Locate a trigger point or adhesion. Test the area by applying friction. If it feels deeper or no progress is made, proceed with this technique.

2. Use a fist, palm, forearm, elbow, or knee (depending on the size of the surface) to press into the area that is having difficulty releasing. Stop when your partner begins to feel pain. Hold this area until all pain is gone and they feel only pressure. Push in a little farther until they feel the "edge" of where that pain signal occurs again. Hold until the pain dissipates to pressure only. Push in one last time until the pain signal appears, and hold until gone.

3. Slowly begin to back the pressure off the area in a rocking or circular friction–type motion. You will notice this area may go from white to red due to having pushed blood flow out and the blood rushing back into the area, making it important to slowly work your way back out of the area.

TRIGGER POINT WITH CIRCULAR FRICTION

This popular neuromuscular technique is a form of deep tissue massage that provides a gentle release of trigger points and adhesions.

1. Locate the trigger point, and use gentle friction in a circular manner.

2. You will notice over time that the area will break down and the adhesion disperse.

SCAR TISSUE RELEASE

We are a lot more vulnerable with our partners than we are with our massage therapist. There are also a lot of areas that may contain scar tissue that a massage therapist may not be able to work on, depending on varying state laws. Scars are made of collagen fiber, just like fascia, and respond to massage. They may or may not be sensitive to touch. The more that you touch the area, the less sensitive it should become.

1. Friction over the scar vertically. Friction over the scar vertically from the opposite direction.

2. Friction over the scar horizontally. Friction over the scar horizontally from the opposite direction.

3. Continue to move back and forth over the scar at as many different angles as possible.

ACTIVE RELEASE TECHNIQUE

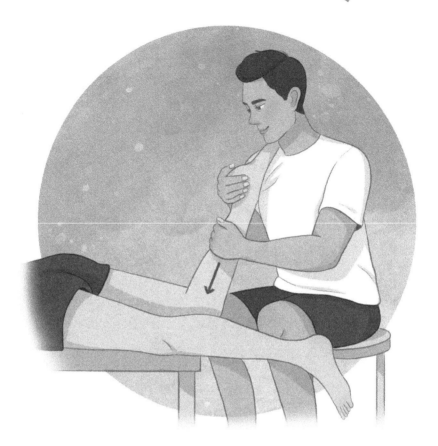

An active release technique involves having your partner engage the muscle group that is bothering them to contract it to its shortest length, to trick the muscle into relaxing.

1. Instruct your partner to do the action of the muscle. Bend your leg, for example.

2. Have them hold it while you squeeze or compress the area while taking a deep breath. Repeat 3 times.

PIN AND STRETCH

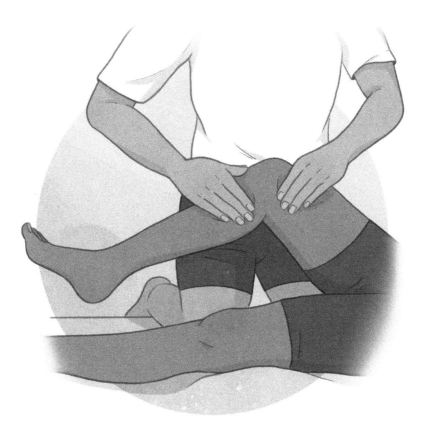

This technique is similar to Active Release (page 68); however, instead of having the partner complete the action, they remain relaxed while you move the body part through the action.

1. While your partner remains relaxed, move the body part through the normal range of motion. If there seems to be an area that grabs or doesn't want to move freely back into position, then compress the area with your hand or fist.

2. Push on the muscle, frictioning it as you stretch it. Bend the body part back. Repeat this until the area seems to loosen.

THUMB ROLLING

1. Hold on to the body part with your thumbs pointed toward each other.

2. Press the thumbs into the tissue while going in opposite directions, so one thumb goes up and one goes down.

FIST HEEL

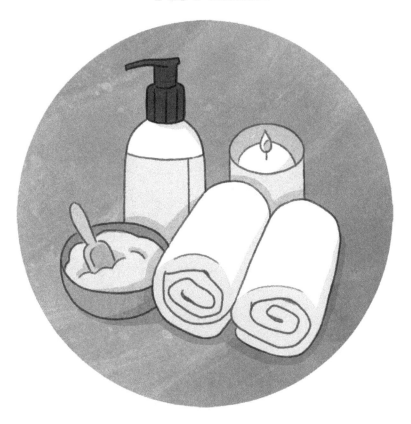

Make a fist. Push into your partner's tissue, rolling your fist down your fingers to the heel of your hand.

TWISTY FISTS

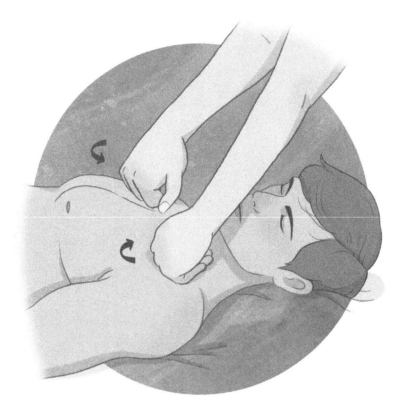

Make a fist with each hand, and twist each fist into the surface of the skin, rotating in opposite directions.

Ayurveda

Ayurveda is a healing and health maintenance system that began in India. It addresses the mind, body, and spirit by achieving balance through a proper diet, exercise, and maintenance of emotional health. In Ayurveda, the world is made up of the five great elements—space, air, fire, water, and earth. There are also associated times and seasons, much like the Chinese medicine wheel. These five elements make up our bodily composition, or "dosha." The three doshas are "vata," "pitta," and "kapha." Whenever the doshas are out of balance, they may affect not only ourselves, but also our relationships with our partners. Abhyanga is an Ayurvedic form of oil massage that can help the doshas reachieve balance. By recognizing the traits of the doshas in our relationships, we can adjust our massage to help achieve balance so our relationships may flourish. Nourishing ourselves first may even cure animosity within our relationships that we knowingly cause ourselves.

Vata, made of space and air, is characterized by a thin light frame, delicate digestion, cold hands and feet, irregular sleep patterns, and dry skin and hair. Typically, these people move and talk very quickly, resist routine, and love new experiences. When they are balanced, they adapt quickly and are excitable and highly energetic. They love adventure and meeting new people. They are spontaneous individuals; they think outside the box, and are very outspoken. When they are out of balance, they may frequently be late, anxious, fearful, and full of worry, often blaming themselves. This may cause them to be confused, sad, or depressed. They may struggle with forgetting to eat, constipation, gas, and bloating.

They may struggle to finish projects due to a lack of focus, have an overactive mind, constantly chatter, and struggle with insomnia. They can benefit from a massage with a heavier heated oil, such as sesame seed, almond, castor, or avocado. Adding a warming, grounding, earthy, and sweet oil such as vanilla, rose, clove, orange, bergamot, basil, geranium, patchouli, vetiver, fir needle, tangerine, or ylang ylang can add to the experience. Warm, soothing, soft, and calming music can help them increase depleted energy. Their massage should be very nourishing and nurturing, to counteract any depletion in their nature.

Pitta is made up of fire and water to create transformation. These people are often of medium build. They have a strong digestive system. Their body temperature runs warm. They are of sharp intellect and learn quickly. They communicate very directly with their speech and actions, making them intense but courageous. They love routine and may be considered perfectionists. When they are balanced, they are friendly, talented leaders, and have warm personalities. When they are out of balance, their demand for perfection may make them aggressive, angry, blameful, sad, depressed, excessively critical, irritable, judgmental, mean, and impatient. Imbalance can cause headaches, migraines, indigestion, heartburn, inflammation, and skin rashes. Pitta benefits the most from light, cooling massage oils like coconut, olive, sunflower, safflower, or ghee with sweet, cooling, or calming oils such as rose, sandalwood, jasmine, fennel, spearmint, lemon, lavender, lime, lemongrass, tea tree, or neroli. Pitta can benefit from calm, cool, steady music with sweet sounds. Pitta types need a slower massage to balance out their quick, fiery nature.

Kapha is made of earth and water. These people may be more heavyset with hearty stamina and rarely get sick. This may be due to the fact that they get deep, sound sleep. They have a cooler body temperature. Typically, they have smooth skin and thick hair, and are solid, stable, smooth, steady, slow-moving, easygoing, methodical, sweet, and caring, and enjoy routine. In balance, they are calm, consistent, content, loyal, steady, strong, and supportive. When they are out of balance, they have a tendency to be attached, complacent, dull, greedy, needy, and overly protective. When they become immobile, they have a tendency to withdraw and overeat when sad or depressed. They also have a tendency to become congested and experience sinus and allergy problems when out of balance. Kapha needs invigorating; use heating oils such as mustard, jojoba, or safflower. They may be paired with essential oils that are invigorating, warming, and uplifting, and spices such as clove, eucalyptus, rosemary, cinnamon, peppermint, wintergreen, grapefruit, ginger, lemon, lime, and rose. Kapha needs stimulating, warming, robust, cheerful, and active music during a massage. A quicker stimulating massage will help relieve the stagnation that causes congestion within the body.

In Ayurveda, the scalp and the feet are highly regarded, because all the meridians run through the scalp and the feet. Here are a few variations of Ayurvedic massage traditions to try at home with your significant other:

SHIRODHARA

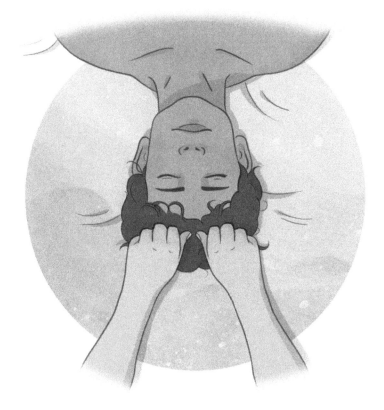

Shirodhara is the gentle application of hot oil to the third eye—just above and between the eyebrows. Once the oil drips into the hair, it is massaged into the scalp. This can potentially be messy. Consider putting down plastic, such as a trash bag, to protect surfaces. At our office, I put the trash bag under the sheets and funnel them back into a bucket to catch the excess oil.

1. Heat the oil until it's warm to the touch but won't burn.

2. Tilt your partner's head back so that the oil won't drain into their face and will go instead into the container that you plan to catch it in. Slowly pour the oil back and forth over the forehead, allowing the oil to drain back over the head through the hair. Be aware of the eyes.

3. When all the oil is gone, compress the receiver's forehead. Do some circling over the temples before continuing the circling motions through the hair. Twist the hair together to drain out the oil. Use a towel to remove excess oil.

INDIAN SCALP MASSAGE

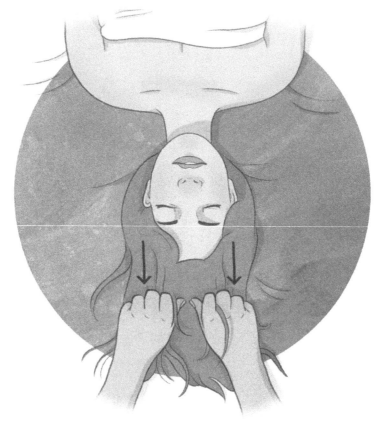

1. Begin the massage with compressions with the palm of your hand to help your partner adjust to the pressure. You may wish to incorporate some rubbing movements into this.

2. Start to use your fingertips instead of the whole palm to compress areas of the head. Tap the scalp gently with your fingertips in a drumlike motion.

3. When you tire of tapping the head, begin to knead the scalp with your fingertips. Transition into small pulling movements with the hair to loosen the scalp.

4. End by running your hands through your partner's hair.

ABHYANGA

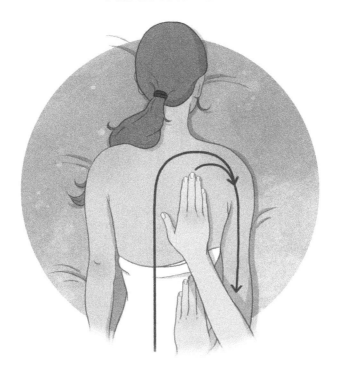

Abhyanga is a massage personalized to the dosha that uses long repetitive movements in odd numbers to stimulate the body. Assess your partner's dosha using a quiz or the information on page 73 regarding the composition of doshas and balances and imbalances. There are many quizzes for this available online. Use the result to choose your oils and to plan your massage. Kapha will need a quicker massage due to their slower tendency. Pitta will need a slower massage to slow down their fiery nature, and vata will need a more nurturing massage to ground them from their air and space elements.

1. Using long, flowing effleurage strokes, work up and down each side of the spine for an odd number of strokes. Starting at the top of the hips, friction the tissue off of each side of the spine all the way to the top of the back and repeat for an odd number of strokes.

2. Use long, flowing effleurage strokes down each arm for an odd number of strokes. Then use large effleurage down the legs for an odd number of strokes.

CONTINUES

3. Have your partner roll over. Use long effleurage strokes down the legs for an odd number of strokes. Use long effleurage strokes down both arms. Apply the oil to the abdomen and use circling on the abdomen.

4. Next, effleurage the face, avoiding the eyes. End with a scalp massage with lots of circling. Lighten your touch as you end the massage and take your hands away.

INDIAN FOOT MASSAGE

The Indian foot massage is considered sacred because of a cultural belief that the meridians, as well as the chakras (which bare the soul), are located in the soles of the feet, where they all converge. This massage helps balance both.

1. Rub your hands with warm oil.

2. Start with the right foot. Gently rub in small circular motions over the soles of the feet and the ankles. Apply pressure with your thumb on the top of the foot in the groove where it meets the shin. Drag your thumb from this spot to the end of each toe, starting with the big toe before going to the next toe. Interlace your fingers with the toes and move in a circular motion.

3. Next, drag your thumb from the end of each toe to the heel of the toe on the sole of the foot, starting with the pinky toe and ending with the big toe. Make a fist and twist the fist into the sole and arch of the foot. Pull each toe.

4. Repeat with the left foot.

5. Soak the feet in a tub of warm water and Epsom salts for 5 to 10 minutes.

Chakras

Chakras are considered to be part of traditional Indian medicine. A chakra is a spinning vortex of energy that lies along the midline of the body. It is closely related to consciousness as well as endocrine glands. Achieving balance within the endocrine system, which produces hormones, is associated with youthful vitality.

ROOT CHAKRA is located at the base root or perineum, associated with the color red, the spinal column, legs, kidneys, colon, gonads, and ovaries, and basic survival needs like shelter and security.

SACRAL CHAKRA is associated with the sacrum and adrenal glands, and represents pleasure, emotional balance, and sexuality. It is linked to the color orange and the reproductive organs, prostate, and bladder.

SOLAR PLEXUS CHAKRA is associated with the color yellow and is located by the belly button. It deals with issues of willpower and assertion and supports the pancreas as well as the liver and stomach.

HEART CHAKRA is associated with green or pink and the thymus gland, which regulates the immune system. This chakra represents love, acceptance, compassion, and intuitiveness.

THROAT CHAKRA is associated with the color blue, the thyroid, and parathyroid glands. It represents communication, creativity, truth, and reliability. The body parts are the hypothalamus, throat, and mouth.

THIRD EYE CHAKRA is deep purple and is located in the center of the brain, at a point between the eyes and just above the ears. It represents wisdom, imagination, intuition, and an ability to analyze and perceive truth in the world. The associated body parts are the pituitary gland, the nose, the ears, and the pineal gland.

CROWN CHAKRA is the only chakra found outside the physical body; it is located just above the crown of the head in what is considered the "spiritual body." It is associated with higher consciousness, pure unconditional life, and a state of pure being.

Craniosacral

Craniosacral therapy makes an attempt to alter the central nervous system through the movement of cerebrospinal fluid, cranial sutures, the orbits, the palates, cranial nerves, cranial bones, joints, teeth, sutural ligaments, the vertebrae, the sacrum, the coccyx, and the pelvis. In this therapy the giver attempts to make contact with the transmission of brainwave activity and influence the flow and production of cerebrospinal fluid. Traditional "listening stations" include the tops and bottoms of the feet, the calves, the thighs, the hips, the abdomen, thoracic outlet and inlet, the arms and hands, the neck, the base of the skull, and the calvarium.

VAULT HOLD

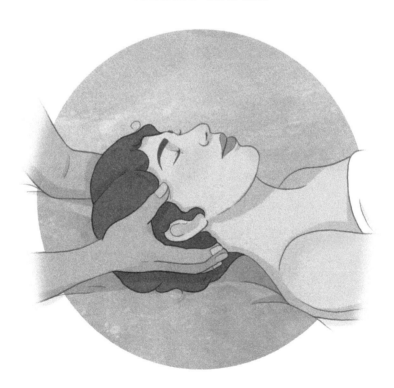

1. Sit behind your partner's head with them lying faceup.
2. Cradle their head with their ears between your third and fourth fingers.

CRANIAL RHYTHM

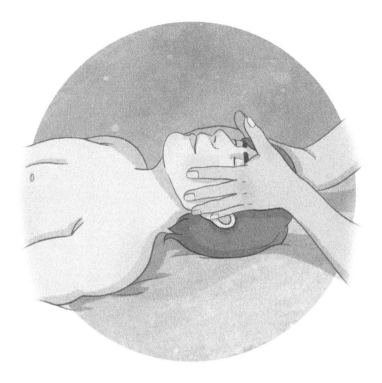

1. Perform the Vault Hold (opposite).

2. Try to palpate the cranial rhythm for 1 minute. Straighten your arms and begin to feel the motion in your arms and chest. Try to "ride" with the rhythm and move your hands with the motion.

PROPRIOCEPTIVE PERCEPTION

1. Have your partner hold their hands out palms up. Rest your hands on their hands with a light touch.

2. Rotate your hands to create a "cranial respiratory impulse." Close your eyes and feel the motion in your forearms and elbows.

3. Try to see what kind of subtle motions you can feel.

STILL POINT HOLD AT FEET

1. Have your partner lie faceup. Cup both of their heels gently. Mold your hands to their heels without grasping them.

2. Feel in your arms for craniosacral movement as it rotates the feet. "Ride" the rhythm until it stops.

OCCIPITAL DECOMPRESSION

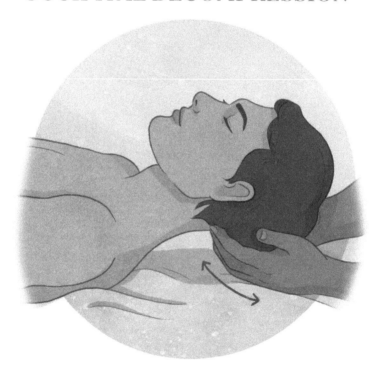

1. Have your partner lie faceup. Cup their head in your hands. Curl your fingers and hook into the space under the head and neck. Allow the head to relax until you feel a release.

2. Gently traction the head from the spine. Repeat this traction until you reach the dural tube—the membrane that surrounds the spinal cord.

Acupressure

Acupressure points are located along the meridians we discussed in part 1 (page 11) and are found using anatomical and bony landmarks. The distance between points is called "cun." Each cun is the size of the receiver's own thumb knuckle. Each acupressure point has the diameter of a nickel to a quarter. Acupressure points can be stimulated using your fingers, magnetic pellets on a piece of tape, ear seeds, or even a mini massager. Magnets or ear seeds may remain in place for up to 8 hours. The difference between acupressure and acupuncture is that acupuncture uses a small needle to stimulate these points. Firm pressure is required to activate the point. Most points require 5 to 10 minutes of concentrated time, depending on what is being treated and the degree of illness. The effects of acupressure are not usually felt immediately. Typically, it takes about an hour before you feel the effects. Acupressure can be done to help regulate bodily function. Signs that an acupressure point is being properly stimulated include itching, tingling, numbness, aching, and warmth.

Acupressure Points

Relieve common tensions and discomforts with these acupressure points.

LARGE INTESTINE 4: This point lies in the space between the thumb and index finger. Do not stimulate while pregnant, as this is considered an induction point. Helps with allergies, arm pain, cold and flu, hand pain, headaches, hives, sinus congestion, and nosebleed.

JIA BI: These points are located on either side of the nose where your glasses would sit. These points are great for sinus headaches.

GALLBLADDER 20, 21: These points are located at the base of the skull where it meets the neck. Bend fingers and hook into the space on either side of the spine to find these.

REN 12, 13, 14: Good for migraines in the center of the forehead. These points lie below the sternum and the rib cage in the center of the abdomen above the belly button.

SPLEEN 6: Used for hormone balance, PMS, water retention, anemia, anxiety, headache, infertility, insomnia, labor induction, and uterine prolapse. Located on the inner ankle 1 hand width above the ankle bone behind the shinbone.

LIVER 3: Notably the best point for treating stress, PMS, insomnia, and depression. Located on the foot between the big toe and second toe.

HEART 7: This point is in the crease line of your wrist. It is in line with the space between your ring and pinky finger. It calms the mind, and helps regulate heartbeat, anxiety, insomnia, and irritability.

PERICARDIUM 6: This point is located 2 points above the wrist crease in the center of the forearm. Aids with anxiety, stomach upset, hiccups, insomnia, irregular heartbeat, and nausea.

KIDNEY 3: The most commonly used point on the kidney meridian. Located behind the inner ankle bone. Also helpful for tinnitus, asthma, insomnia, and urinary issues.

KIDNEY 6: Calms the mind, and ties directly into hot flashes, insomnia, uterine prolapse, and swelling. Located 1 finger width above the inner ankle bone.

STOMACH 36: Located between the two bones of the lower legs. Can be found by bending the knee and moving your fingers up the shin until you find where the two bones meet. Has the potential to help with belching, fullness, diarrhea, constipation, nausea, poor appetite, vomiting, fatigue, asthma, cough, shortness of breath, allergies, colds, and flu.

PLUCKING

Locate the area where the acupressure point is found. Pull the tissue back. Then push the tissue forward. Then pull the tissue back, plucking it like a guitar string.

CIRCULAR FRICTION

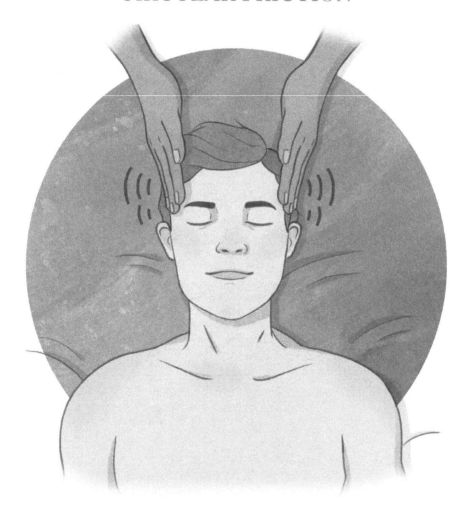

Locate the area where the acupressure point is found. Use your fingertips or a knuckle in a circling motion to stimulate an acupressure point for 1 minute.

TAPPING

Locate the area where the acupressure point is. Drum your fingers over the area one at a time or simultaneously.

Reflexology

Reflexology is an ancient form of Chinese medicine based on the belief that there are correlating points for the organs and parts of the body in the hands, feet, and ears. This is plausible due to the correlation of meridian lines running through the points connecting and regulating energies and activities. These lines in the feet that run longitudinally (or lengthwise) are called zones. In traditional Chinese medicine, the body is divided into the upper jaw, middle jaw, and lower jaw. The foot is also divided up this way. In addition, the side of the instep of the foot and the large toe coordinates with the spine as well as the chakras that lie along the spine.

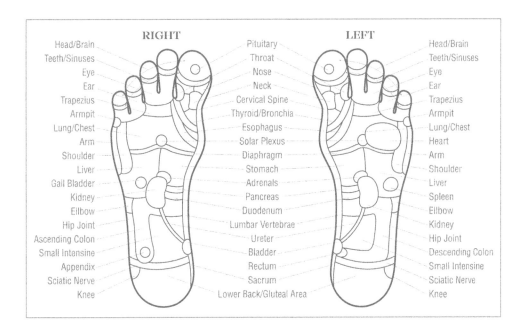

DUCK PECK TECHNIQUE

I learned the duck peck technique from Janet Wolf Blevins, a mentor and a fellow continuing education instructor trained in acupressure and various forms of Ayurveda and Chinese medicine. This method protects the fingers and particularly the thumb from strain and injury during reflexology. Alternatively, you may wish to use tools to friction and compress areas of the foot.

1. Bend the thumb at the first joint. This creates the duck's bill.

2. Use the tip of the bent thumb to press into the area of the foot you wish to activate. You may "peck," hold, or apply friction this way with your thumb.

BENDING THE JOINTS

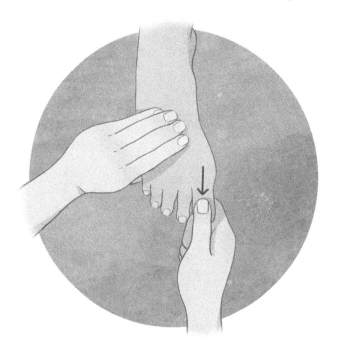

This is a fine movement that allows for the release of gas in the toe joints and the breaking up of any waste stored there due to gravity.

Start with the large toes. Bend the toe at each joint until it moves easily and no longer clicks.

SPREADING THE TOES

This is a great way to stretch the toes.

1. Put your fingers in between all of your partner's toes.

2. Work the fingers slowly and gently down until the toes are interlocked with your hand. Move the toes toward the ankle and back toward the heel, stretching the top and the bottom of the foot.

BREAKING BREAD OR CHUCKING

This movement helps break up the energy blockages in the toes.

1. Grasp two toes side by side. Push one toe up while pushing the other down gently.

2. Repeat on all toes.

Tantra

Contrary to common belief, tantric massage is not necessarily about having sex. Tantra as well as erotic massage styles are really about connecting with your partner through mind, spirit, heart, and body. This stronger spiritual connection can then support the physical relationship between lovers. It builds trust and loving energy between partners.

One of the most important ways of preparing for tantric massage involves making uninterrupted time for this massage. Freeing yourselves of distractions, outside noise, and interruptions is important for creating a proper exchange of energy between you and your partner. This should be a time of focusing on what you admire about your partner, and not judging their imperfections, to get the positive energy flowing between both parties. Tantra involves stimulating the seven chakras along the spine to free any blocked energies. The zones stimulated are called erogenous zones. They run along the governing and conception vessel meridians where the flow of chi may be disrupted by stress, illness, or fatigue, throwing yin and yang out of balance.

TANTRIC MASSAGE TECHNIQUES

Men and women have different erogenous zones. For women, these are located along the chakra lines along the center of the body: at the top of the head, above the top lip, below the bottom lip, down both sides of the sternum, the center of the abdomen, along the bikini line, 1 hand width on either side of the lower back, and where the lower back dimples. For men, these are located at the tip of the head, the upper lip, bottom lip, along both sides of the sternum, below the belly button, where the groin connects to the upper thigh, the base of the neck, and at the sacral bone in the lower back.

GLIDING HAND

1. Run your hands down the center of the body from the head to the midsection.

2. Pay close attention to the erogenous areas mentioned above.

FEATHERING

Using the tips of your fingers, trace the lines related to the erogenous zones mentioned on page 90.

TRACING

Using your fingertips, trace your partner's body from the top of their head to their hip and waist area.

1. Have your partner lie faceup. Run your fingers through your partner's hair, making contact with the top of the center of the skull.

2. Glide your fingertips from the top of the head down the center of the face to the top lip.

3. Press for 5 seconds lightly on the top lip and then outline the lips moving to the bottom lip, pressing and holding again for 5 seconds.

4. Sweep your hands down the neck, locating the breastbone, or sternum, in the center of the chest.

5. Sweep your fingertips off each side of the sternum, moving outward toward the armpits, returning to the center of the body, and working your way down the torso each time.

6. Run your hands up from the inside of the upper leg out toward the glutes.

7. Gently hook your hands under the lower back, raking your hands from the spine to the hips. Then hook your hands under your partner at the waist and pull your hands from the hips to the neck.

8. End by gently cradling the head and neck, massaging with fingertips.

Part 3

LET THE MASSAGE BEGIN

Everyone loves a good massage. Now it's time to get acclimated and comfortable with your partner through massaging each other. There are so many reasons and occasions for a good massage. It can happen on any typical day, or it can happen on a special day like a birthday. The great thing about massaging your significant other at home is that it is a great gift that you can enjoy together with minimal costs. It can be as fancy or as relaxed as you wish. In this section we will begin to bring together the pieces that you have learned about massage thus far. Let's combine these techniques from all over the world to help meet your partner's specific needs.

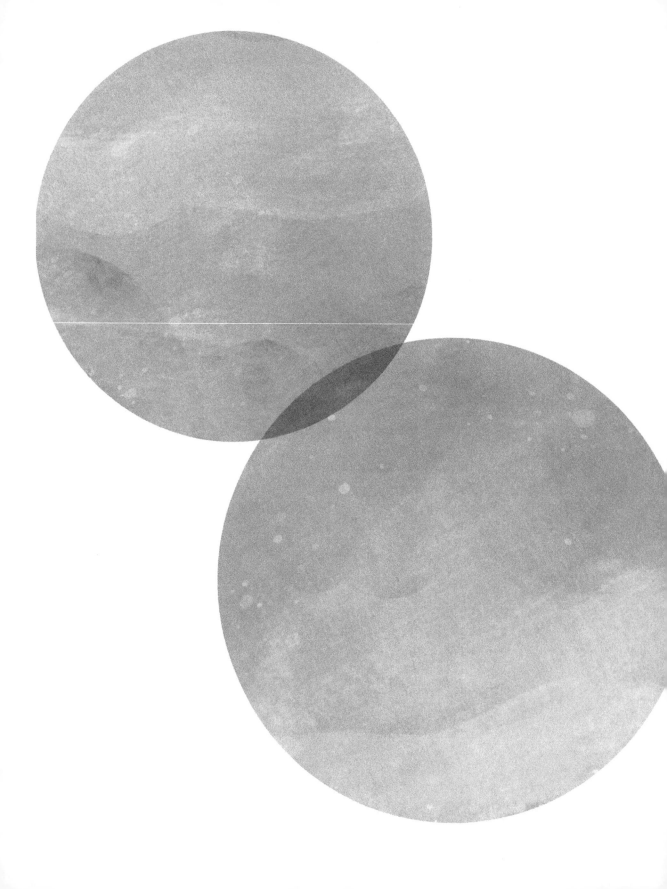

Chapter 6
The Whole Body Awaits

Our bodies make up one amazing system, with each part performing a vital task and functioning in a unique way. Because our muscle fibers run differently in different parts of the body, a massage technique that felt right in one area may not feel the same on another part of the body. This is what makes giving a massage an adventure and an opportunity to attune to your partner's body, mind, and unique way of feeling sensations. As you practice this sensitivity, you'll reach your ultimate goal of relief, romance, or bonding. In this chapter, we will break down techniques for each area of the body.

Head and Face

The face and head are often neglected during massages. Don't underestimate the joy and invigoration of a good scalp or face massage. These areas often carry a lot of tension and can relax a great deal during a massage. Even the delicate features of the face can be gently massaged. As always, avoid heavy pressure over the eyes, the temples, and the nose. Surprisingly, a lot can be done with the head to provide you with great relief. All of these methods will be done with your partner lying faceup. Avoid using a heavy oil or lotion on the face, which may cause breakouts. A good option for this may be grape-seed, coconut, or jojoba oil. Small amounts of essential oils such as tea tree, frankincense, lavender, and eucalyptus can provide various therapeutic effects on the head and face.

ANTI-AGING FACIAL MASSAGE

The lymphatic system relies on musculoskeletal movement to move fluid along. Other than talking, chewing, and making facial expressions, our face does little moving. This method can help move the lymph in the face to reduce puffiness.

1. Sweep the fingers up from the eyebrows to the hairline 3 to 5 times.

2. Next, sweep the fingers on the outside of the nose to the jaw 3 to 5 times.

3. Start at the corners of the mouth and sweep up toward the ears 3 to 5 times.

4. Next, sweep the fingers from the jaw lightly down the neck to the collarbone.

TMJ MASSAGE

Temporomandibular joint disorder can manifest in severe head, ear, and face pain. Relaxing the muscles that cause strain on the joint may ease discomfort.

1. Slide your fingers from the ear to the cheek, working your way down the cheek toward the jaw.

2. Then begin to massage the cheek in a circular motion using gentle pressure.

3. Continue to do this while instructing your partner to open and close their mouth and shift their jaw from left to right.

SINUS MASSAGE

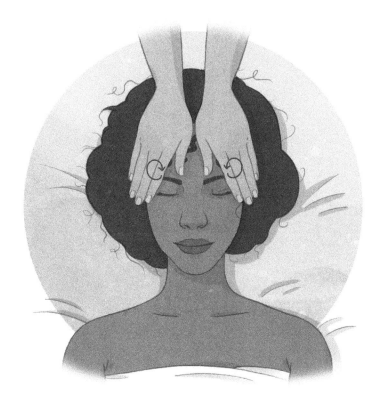

In times of sickness and stuffiness, consider using this method to help your partner breathe easier, whether suffering from sinus headache, seasonal allergies, or even a cold.

1. Place your fingers above the eyebrows.
2. Make small circles with your fingers from the start of the eyebrows to the temples 3 times.
3. Pinch the bridge of the nose, holding for 15 seconds.
4. Sweep down the sides of the nose toward the corner of the mouth. Repeat 3 times.
5. Make small circles below the check but above the teeth.

STIMULATING SCALP MASSAGE

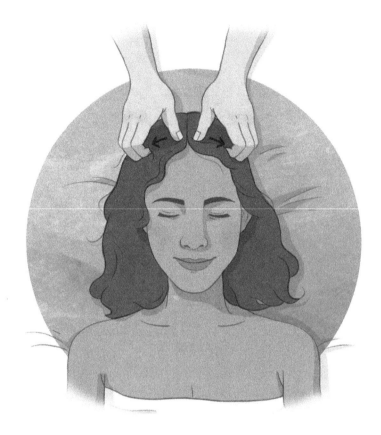

An invigorating scalp massage may release tension that causes head-aches, as well as help stimulate hair growth.

1. Place both hands on top of the head with fingers pointed to the ears.

2. Knead gently and make small circles throughout the hair, occasionally compressing areas of the scalp using your thumbs.

A REAL CLENCHER

This technique is great to use for clenching of the jaw, affecting the head, face, and scalp.

1. Put your hands on top of the head with the backs of the wrists together and the fingers pointing toward the ears.

2. Push your hands downward, raking the fingertips through the hair and down the sides of the face. Repeat this as you move across the top of the head.

3. Next, locate the area above the ears with your fingertips. Massage and compress the area in a circular motion.

4. Move down toward the jaw, sweeping downward.

JAW DROPPER

This technique may aid with jaw- and smiling-related pain, which takes away from enjoying time with your significant other.

1. Glide your hands or flat palms gently down the side of each cheek from cheekbone to jaw.

2. Have your partner open their mouth, and repeat this motion.

3. Ask your partner to open their mouth and shift their jaw to the right. Next, allow your partner to close their mouth, and gently massage the cheek with effleurage.

4. Glide your hands down the side of each cheek.

5. Repeat step 3 on the left side.

EFT TAPPING

EFT tapping is a method used to activate acupressure lines and points in the body. It stimulates the body's flow of energy by tapping these points with the tips of the fingers to disrupt energy flow and create distraction that may help with energy, anxiety, or concentration. Each point can be tapped for as long as it feels comfortable.

1. Tap your fingers on the top of the middle of the head.

2. Tap your fingers on the ends of the eyebrows closest to the nose.

3. Tap your fingers at the outside corner of the eyes.

4. Tap your fingers under the eyes where we get "bags."

5. Tap your fingers under the center of the nose above the top lip.

6. Tap your fingers at the center of the chin.

DECOMPRESS

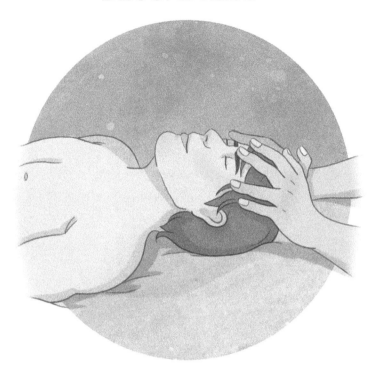

The face holds a lot of tension, as well as being the location for anxiety acupressure points along the brow between the eyes.

1. Gently use your two index fingers to glide over the area above the nose between the eyebrows. Pinch the area that lies between the eyes above the nose.

2. Moving gently, make light circles over the forehead using the fingertips of both hands. Move gently down to the temples with small slow circles.

3. Gently compress the forehead for 5 to 10 seconds by pressing down on the forehead with steady, even pressure.

4. End by lightly running your fingers down each side of the nose.

EAR MOOD LIFTER

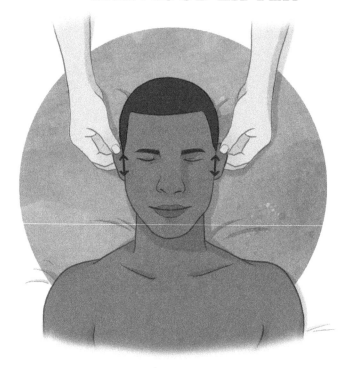

There are many acupressure points in the ear that help improve mood.

1. Gently pinch the outside of the ears.

2. Moving up and down the outside edge of the ear, hold each spot for 5 to 10 seconds.

3. Work your way around the inside of the ear where the inner fold is, as you did the outside.

EARACHE RELIEF

Congestion that causes the ears to feel full is no joke. Try this method to help open the ear canals during allergy season.

1. Massage the area behind both ears with your fingertips, making small circles.

2. Sweep the fingers from under the earlobe to the square of the jaw 3 times.

3. Then gently pinch the earlobes, tugging them down and back. Repeat as desired.

FACE-LIFTING MASSAGE

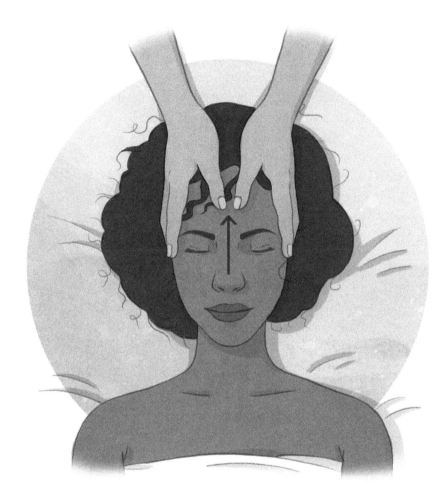

This technique works against gravity, which causes wrinkles and fine lines.

1. Interlace your fingers under your partner's chin, tilting the head back.

2. Rake the fingers up either side of the chin, up the face to the head, 3 to 5 times.

3. Touch your fingers together on either side of the nose, and sweep them to the front of the small raised divot in front of the ear 3 to 5 times.

4. Put all five fingers on the eyebrows and rake them upward 3 to 5 times.

Neck

Due to the weight of our head, the neck can often experience strain and discomfort. It consists of lots of short and long thin muscles all working together to balance the weight of a bowling ball. The neck can turn the head left, right, forward, backward, and side to side. Within the neck you have the carotid artery. It may be palpable when sliding the fingers down the neck and under the jaw. In the event that you begin to feel a heartbeat, you will want to move off this spot. The brachial plexus, a bundle of nerves that runs down the arm, is also located here and will result in sharp pain when irritated. Although massaging the neck can help reduce headache-related pain, when you massage, typically you want to massage down toward the body away from the brain in case of stroke or clotting issues. Always avoid head pressure over the front of the neck. All of the techniques in this section will be performed lying faceup unless specified otherwise.

TRACTIONING THE NECK WITH A TOWEL OR PILLOWCASE

For this technique, you will need a pillowcase or towel.

1. Position the towel or pillowcase under the base of the head, and take each side of the towel into your hands.

2. Lift gently upward. Next, pull the head, stretching to the left so the ear is closing in on the shoulder, and hold for 10 seconds. Then pull it to the right.

3. Turn the head using the towel so the cheek touches the surface your partner is lying on to the left. Then turn it to the right.

GENTLY LOVING SQUEEZE

This method is an easy way to show your partner some quick affection.

1. Make contact with the base of your partner's neck with the webbing between the index finger and thumb.

2. Squeeze and hold.

3. Pull the hand away, gently lessening your grip.

TENSION HEADACHE TAMER

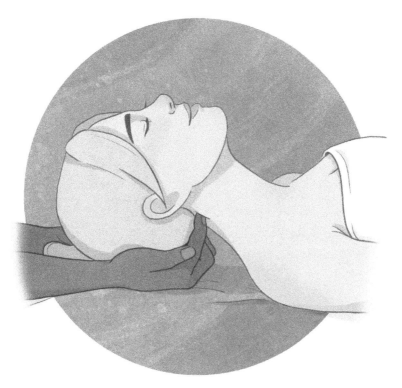

Many people who experience chronic headaches and migraines experience them at the base of the head, where the skull attaches to the neck. Sometimes these types of headaches will refer pain behind the eyes and over the eyebrows into the temples.

1. Run your fingers up the back of the neck toward the base of the skull. Hook and push in between the neck and the skull.

2. Scrunch your fingers up and down, feeling for areas of tightness.

3. Hold areas that feel tight while instructing your partner to take deep breaths until the muscles relax.

LATERAL NECK STRETCH

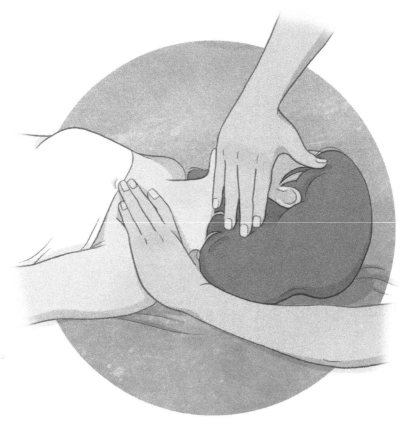

1. Use one hand to anchor the shoulder down so it doesn't move.

2. Use the opposite hand to press into the side of the head.

3. Gently push the head and neck to the opposite side so the ear is almost to the shoulder, stretching the neck. Do not strain the neck. Check in with your partner to make sure you are not overstretching the neck.

4. Return the head back to the center in the neutral position. Repeat on the other side.

STRETCH, COMPRESS, AND FRICTION FOR NECK PAIN

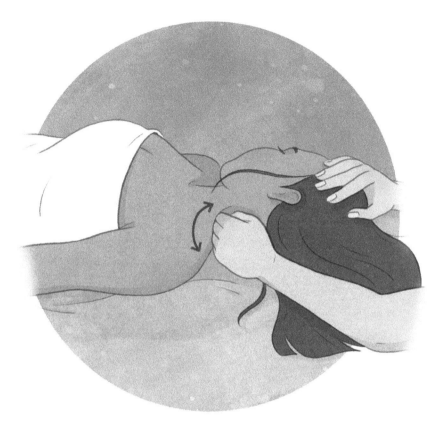

Neck pain is common in those who regularly work at a computer or desk. If this describes your partner's daily work activities, they may enjoy this routine.

1. Gently push the head and neck to one side so the ear is almost to the shoulder, stretching the neck. Use one hand to anchor the shoulder, and use the other hand to press into the side of the head.

2. Remove the hand from the shoulder, and make a fist. Run the fist down the neck from the base of the head to the shoulder, stopping to compress the area when it feels tight or stuck.

3. Repeat on the opposite side of the neck.

CHIN TILT

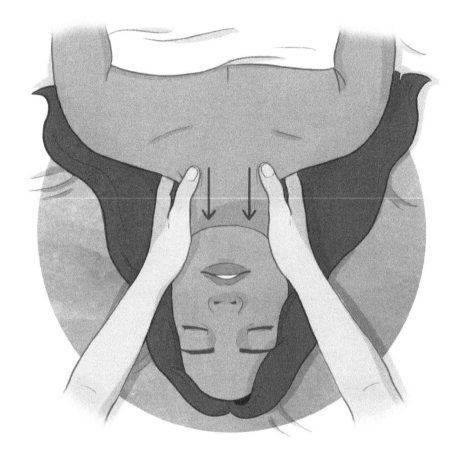

This movement can help stretch the front of the neck.

1. Move both hands up the sides of the neck.
2. Pull the head and chin up and back.

TURN AND FRICTION

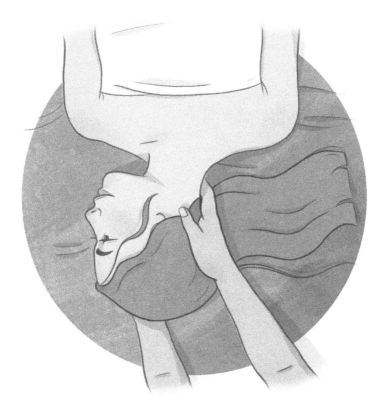

1. Turn the head to one side.

2. Use small circular friction to work your fingers from the base of the skull to the collarbone.

3. Return the neck to the neutral position, and repeat on the other side.

TRACTIONING THE NECK WITH HANDS

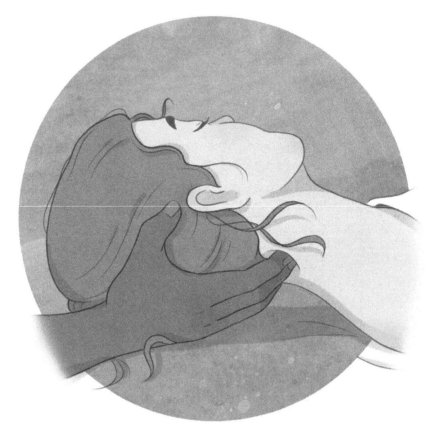

Fight the effects of gravity on the head and neck with this exercise.

Hook your hands under the base of the neck where it meets the head, and gently pull and hold for 5 to 10 seconds.

NECK ROTATIONS

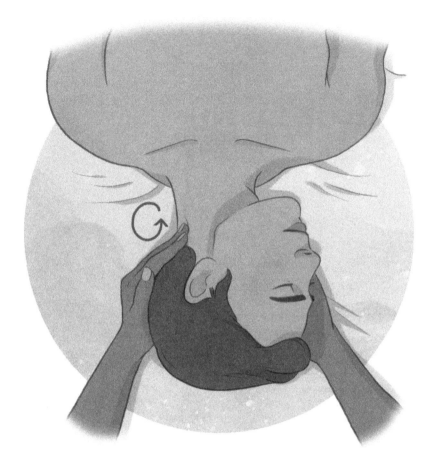

1. Gently cup your partner's head in your hands.

2. Rotate the head around in a circle 3 times. Then gently rotate the head in the opposite direction.

CROSS-HANDED NECK STRETCH

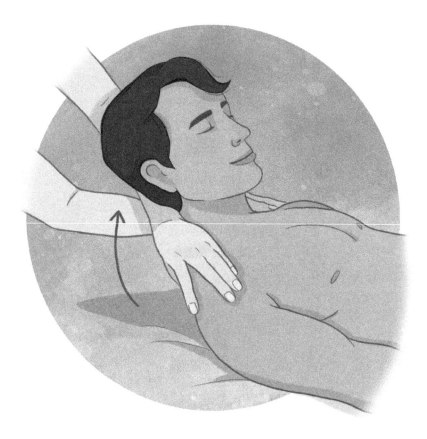

1. Cross your arms, planting each arm firmly on the opposite shoulder.

2. Lift the head slightly to stretch the neck, using your arms for support.

TRAP STRETCH

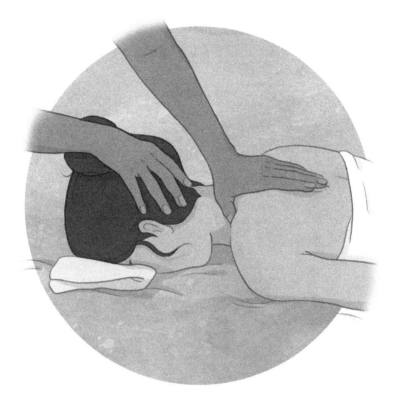

1. Have your partner lie facedown.

2. Hook your finger under the base of the skull. With your other hand, push toward the top of the shoulder, stretching the upper to middle trapezius muscle.

Shoulders

There's nothing like a shoulder massage to take away the weight of the world. The shoulders consist of multiple smaller muscles making up the rotator cuff. The deltoids and pecs both pull on the shoulder joints, causing discomfort and occasional pain. The shoulder joint is a ball-and-socket joint, which means the upper arm can move all the way around the socket. If the fascia builds up in this joint, it can cause the shoulder to lose mobility. This is often called frozen shoulder. The shoulders are highly affected by posture as well as the weight of the chest.

SCAPULA SAVER

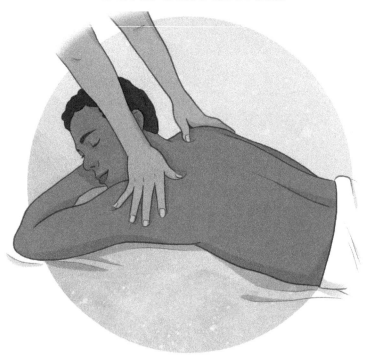

1. Have your partner lie facedown. Run both of your thumbs along the border of their scapula.

2. Whenever you find a knot, compress it with your thumbs or friction over it repeatedly.

SHOULDER PRESS

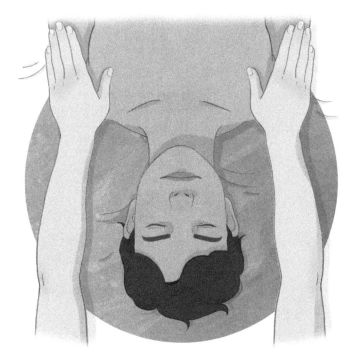

Often our shoulders will round in, causing our upper back to become round. Try this simple technique for relief.

1. Have your partner lie faceup, and place your hands on each shoulder.

2. Press the shoulder straight down onto the work surface, and hold for 10 to 15 seconds.

SCAPULA LIFT

Occasionally, pesky knots will appear rolling under the scapula or shoulder blade. Use this method to get under the shoulder blade.

1. Have your partner lie facedown.

2. Bend the arm behind the back, and press the back of their hand into the middle of their back.

3. Rub the area around the shoulder blade, compressing as needed.

ASSISTED SHOULDER SHRUG

This technique can help free the shoulder when your partner is relaxed and trusting.

1. Have your partner lie facedown with their arms by their side.

2. Place one hand under the shoulder where the chest meets the arm. Rest your other hand on top of the scapula.

3. Lift the bottom hand, picking up the shoulder and moving the shoulder in a forward and backward motion.

MAIN SQUEEZE

This is a great move to help release tension in your partner's neck and shoulders.

1. With your partner sitting or lying down, put one hand on either shoulder. Squeeze and hold gently.

2. Let the tissue slowly melt in your hands on its own.

3. Repeat 3 to 5 times.

SPINE SPREADER

Help improve range of motion and reduce tension in the neck and shoulders with this technique.

1. With your partner sitting or lying facedown, bring the fingers and thumb of one hand together and put them on either side of the spine, beginning at the base of the neck.

2. Push the fingers apart so the hand is open, rubbing the tightness away from the spine. Repeat this motion, walking down the neck and shoulders.

3. Repeat again with the opposite hand.

SHOULDER SMUSHES

Use this technique to relax tight trapezius muscles.

1. Have your partner lie facedown, and stand at your partner's head.
2. Cross your arms and make contact with the base of the neck with the palms of your hands.
3. Push your hands outward toward the shoulders.

SHOULDER SANCTUARY

This technique is enjoyable for those with tight deltoids.

1. Cup both of your hands around the tip of the shoulder and squeeze it.
2. Bend your fingers, raking the fingertips back toward the palm.

LIFTING THE SCAPULA

This technique helps lift the shoulder blade slightly off the rib cage to help get to knots and adhesions more easily.

1. Have your partner lie facedown.
2. Bend their arm to a 90-degree angle, move it behind the back, and press it into the small of the back. You will notice the shoulder blade will pop up.
3. Friction or compress the area, carefully observing tight or "knotty" areas.

SHOULDER STRETCH

This easy stretch targets the chest, shoulders, neck, and lats to increase mobility in the shoulder joints.

1. Have your partner lie facedown, and help them fold both hands behind their head.
2. Slightly pull the elbows back.

Upper Back

The upper back connects the head, neck, and shoulders to the torso. It is often an area of great tension. Times of stress and lack of ease often cause us to elevate our shoulders as if we were wearing them for earrings. The primary muscles of concern in the upper back include the rhomboids, which bring our shoulder blades back toward our spine, and the trapezius muscle, which attaches at the base of the skull, running down the neck, attaching to the shoulders, and coming to a point and attaching at the spine. This area can handle a large amount of pressure.

BREATHE AND HOLD FOR THE BACK

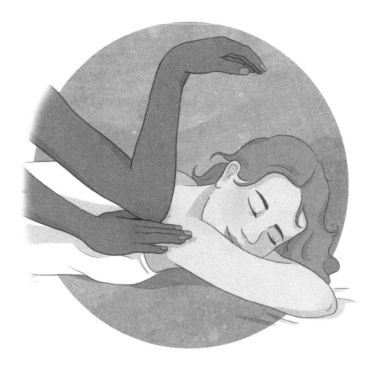

Breathing helps relax areas that are tight and tough to release with fingertip pressure. An alternative method would be to apply circular friction to the adhesed area, roll the skin over the area, or perform petrissage to loosen up any potential adhesions. You may also wish to use an elbow, forearm, or the heel of your foot if you are struggling with pressure.

1. Slowly glide your hands down the sides of the spine, starting at the base of the head and neck and ending at the lower back. Notice any areas of tightness.

2. When you get to an area of tightness or pain, compress the area by stopping on the spot and holding pressure to the area. Instruct the recipient to take a few deep breaths while you hold the area.

3. You will feel the area relax, or the recipient will stop feeling pain. If the area is still tight, but the recipient no longer feels pain, you may apply more pressure until they feel a twinge of discomfort. Instruct them to breathe and communicate with you when they no longer feel pain.

4. Glide your hands back over the area to move fresh blood into the tissue.

5. Repeat over the entire back until pain ceases and tension dissipates.

CUPPING

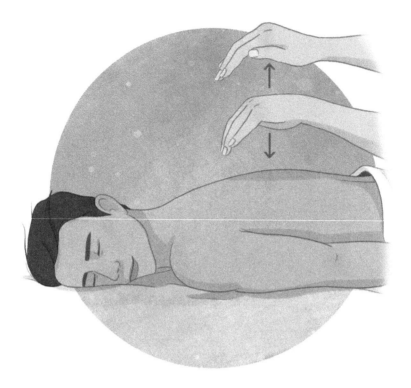

This technique may be a little noisier than some. This is a great technique to perform for chest congestion.

1. Cup your hands.

2. Alternately drum your hands up and down on the upper back. This will make a clapping sound against the skin as you repeat the technique.

3. For more pressure with more developed back muscles, you can use fists instead of cupped hands.

SPINE STRAIGHTENER

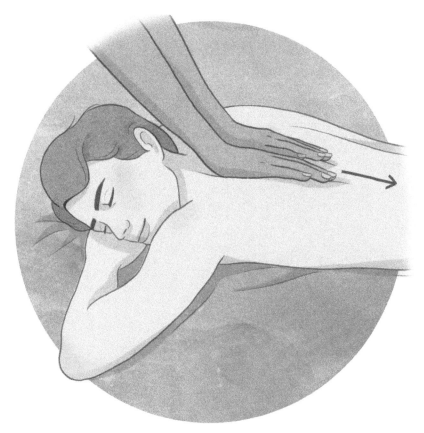

This technique will help relax the muscles lying on either side of the spine.

1. Have your partner lie facedown.

2. Place both of your palms on the back with your fingertips pointing toward your partner's glutes.

3. Push both of your palms down their back, dragging your thumbs along the sides of the spine.

IRONING THE UPPER BACK

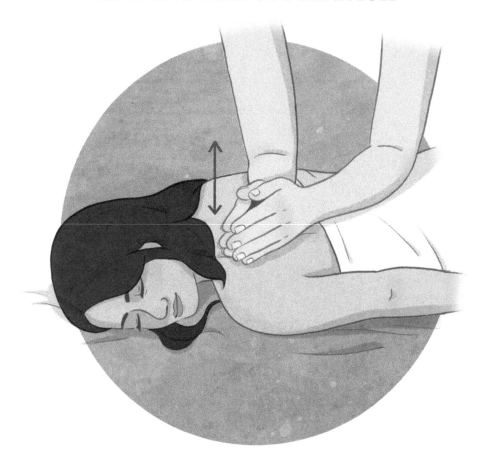

This forearm technique makes relaxing tight upper back muscles a breeze!

1. Have your partner lie facedown.

2. Bend your arms at a 90-degree angle, and gently press down on your partner's back with your broad forearms. Slowly move over the upper back, stopping to hold and compress areas that are tight.

BACKLASH

Oftentimes the muscles in the middle of the back around the spine will become painfully tight, making other techniques difficult due to not being able to work directly over the vertebrae. Try this instead.

1. Locate the vertebrae in the middle of the back and place your hands side by side on one side of the vertebrae, in the groove on either side of the spine.

2. Pull your hands backward, raking them across the tight muscles that hold the spine upright.

3. Repeat on both sides, moving all the way up or down the spine to improve circulation.

A LOVING LIFT

This technique uses your partner's own body weight to help bring more pressure to the upper back.

1. Have your partner lie faceup.

2. Put your hands and arms under their back while instructing your partner to take some deep breaths.

3. Pull your hands from the middle of the back, up the sides of the spine slowly, as your partner relaxes into your hands.

4. Rake the hands up the upper back, traveling up the neck and hooking your fingers under the base of the skull.

5. Repeat 3 times.

WRINGING

This technique helps get deep into the tissue layers.

1. Have your partner lie facedown. Place both of your hands on opposite sides of the body and move them toward each other.

2. Push into the tissue as you reach the place where the opposite hand started.

FASCIAL STRETCH

Use this technique to help stretch the tight fascia of the upper back.

1. Place both hands side by side on the upper back on opposite sides of the spine.

2. Keep one hand planted firmly, pressing into the upper back. With the other hand, press into the back, stretching the fascia using primarily your palm.

3. Repeat with the opposite hands.

CONNECTING STROKE

1. Have your partner lie facedown.

2. Lightly place your hands on the upper back, and slide your hands down to the lower back.

3. Fan the hands out to the hips, and squeeze the hips with both hands.

4. Slide the hands all the way back to where you began.

FANNING

Increase circulation to the upper back with this technique.

1. Slide your hands from the base of the neck out to the tips of the shoulders. Squeeze the shoulders as your hands go over them.

2. Glide the hands back to the base of the neck.

3. Glide the hands over the shoulders just a little bit farther down than you did before. Effleurage back to the base of the neck.

4. Repeat this motion, working all the way down the back.

Lower Back

The lower back can be a very vulnerable area. It is a common source of pain. Two of the primary muscles of the lower back are the quadratus lumborum and latissimus dorsi. The psoas—the long muscle that attaches the lower and upper parts of the body—is a huge source of pain for those who sit for a living. The lower back contains the floating ribs as well as the kidneys. For this reason, heavy pressure on the lower back is not advised to avoid damaging the kidneys and uterus and to avoid breaking a rib. Since lower back pain is often referred from another part of the body, a few techniques in this section involve a range of muscles.

LOVING LOWER LIFT

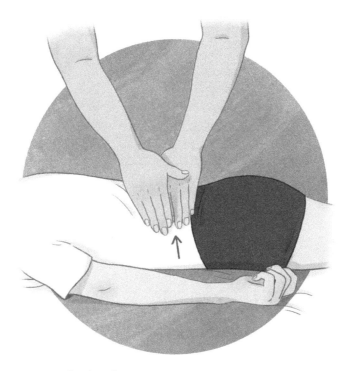

1. Have your partner lie facedown.

2. Place your hands on one side of the lower back. Pull your hands gently across the lower back from one hip to the other. Pull with both hands or hold one hand still while pulling the other hand to the opposite hip.

3. Alternate the hands repeatedly.

MASSAGING THE HAMSTRINGS FOR LOWER BACK PAIN

The hamstrings are some of the strongest muscles in the body. Because of this, they can pull on the back of the pelvis, creating pain in the lower back.

1. Have the recipient lie facedown.

2. Expose the back of the upper leg above the knee. You may or may not wish to expose the glute as well and work on the two areas at the same time.

3. Apply lotion to the back of the leg and/or the glute.

4. Begin by gliding up and down the leg over the area, checking in with your partner about any areas of pain or discomfort.

5. Make two fists or use a forearm to work from right above the back of the knee to compress and glide the tissue over the hamstrings. Do not massage the back of the knee or apply pressure over the back of the knee.

6. Alternatively, you may compress the muscle from the glute to the back of the knee with your shin or even sit on it, if you feel like no change is being made.

MASSAGING THE LOWER BACK

1. Glide your hands from the top of the back down either side of the spine a few times until you reach the top of the hips where they meet the spine. You may also use your fists to glide down.

2. Use vibration to increase circulation to the area.

3. Go to one side of the body, stack your hands, and glide across the lower back where the hip bones join the spine.

4. If you find an area of tightness, you may wish to gently compress above the ribs.

5. Use light circular friction or petrissage over the soft tissue below the ribs, but above the hip bones.

6. End by gently feathering the area.

CROSS-HANDED STRETCH

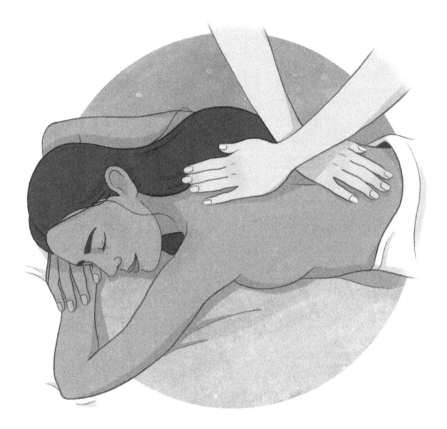

1. Have your partner lie facedown.

2. Cross one arm over the other. Place one hand on the upper middle back and the other on the lower middle back, just above the sacrum.

3. Gently push down and rock back and forth to lengthen the spine.

THE WAVE

1. Have your partner lie facedown.

2. Put one hand on their lower back on the side you are on, and put the other hand on their lower back on the opposite side of their body.

3. Glide your hands to the opposite side, moving up the lower back.

LAT LOVE

1. Have your partner lie facedown. Facing your partner's side, push into their lower back with your forearms.

2. Slowly push into the lower back, sliding your arm closest to their head and neck all the way up to the armpit.

THE HOURGLASS STROKE

1. With your partner lying facedown, place the palms of your hands on their upper back with your fingertips pointed toward the glutes.

2. Run your hands down both sides of the spine. Turn the hands out when you reach the tailbone, and follow your hands out to the sides.

3. Bring your hands back toward the spine. Once you reach the spine, sweep your hands back up the shoulders.

SCOOPS

1. Have your partner lie facedown.

2. Run your hands down either side of their spine.

3. Then make fists. Use your fists and thumbs to push into the lower back.

KNEADING YOU

1. Have your partner lie facedown.

2. Starting at the hip above the buttocks, pick up the tissue with the palm of each hand. Alternate picking up tissue and stroking in a sideways figure-eight motion.

3. Repeat this motion between the hips and armpit on both sides of the body.

KNUCK IT UP

1. Run your hands down the spine, rolling your fingers into either palm to create fists.

2. Roll the knuckles down the spine, pushing to the hips and glutes.

Arms and Hands

The shoulder meets the arm at the deltoid where the humerus bone, which makes up the upper arm, meets the ball-and-socket joint in the shoulder at the rotator cuff. The most notorious muscles of the arm are the biceps and triceps brachii. Both of these muscles cross the elbow to bend the arm. Across the elbow from the humerus is where the ulna and radius are located, with numerous muscles helping turn the wrist and hand, as well as bend the elbow. When muscles on the inside and outside of the elbow experience overuse, people sometimes develop tennis and golfer's elbows, regardless of their choice of leisure activities. Due to typing and texting, these muscles can become tight and sore, pulling on the fingers. The muscles attaching on the forearm run over the 7 tiny carpal bones of the wrist that are bound by a thick layer of fascia referred to as the carpal tunnel. On the other side of this carpal tunnel are lots of smaller bones that form the hand covered by smaller muscles. For massage on the arms and hands, your partner may sit or lie faceup or facedown.

STIMULATING ACUPRESSURE POINTS FOR ANXIETY RELIEF FOR HANDS AND FOREARMS

Follow these steps to stimulate multiple acupressure points in the hand, wrist, and forearm.

1. Squeeze the webbing between the index finger and thumb between your fingers, gliding and rolling over the area multiple times.

2. Next, rub the palm of the hand in small circles where the base of the thumb meets the bottom of the palm.

3. Next, walk your thumbs up the underside of the wrist using small circular friction.

4. Continue to friction the forearm up to the elbow between the bones.

ARTHRITIS RELIEF IN THE HANDS

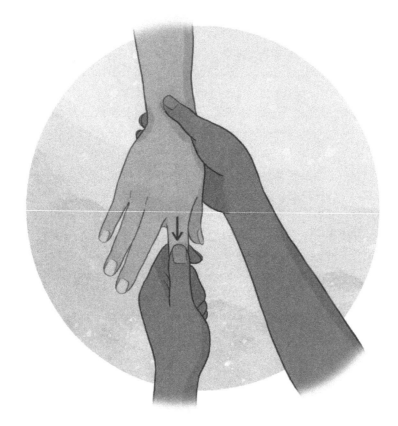

1. Rub the forearms and hands with a gliding motion, returning to the hands.

2. Gently work around each finger, pulling and using small circular friction on each finger.

3. Move the fingers in a circular motion in their joint. Bend each joint in the fingers, frictioning more around those that move less freely.

4. Go to the palm of the hand, and press each finger up and down.

DECOMPRESSING THE HAND AND WRIST

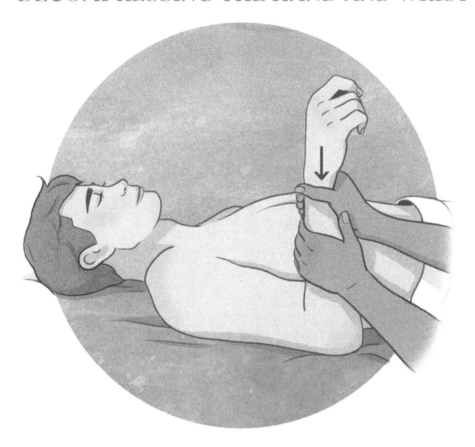

This is a great technique for sore and achy hands due to typing, mechanical work, or carpal tunnel.

1. Have your partner lie on their back and bend their arm to a 90-degree angle.

2. Grasp their wrist with both of your hands at the base of the palm and wrist.

3. Gently massage up and down the forearm, pushing upward into the palm.

WRIST DECOMPRESSION

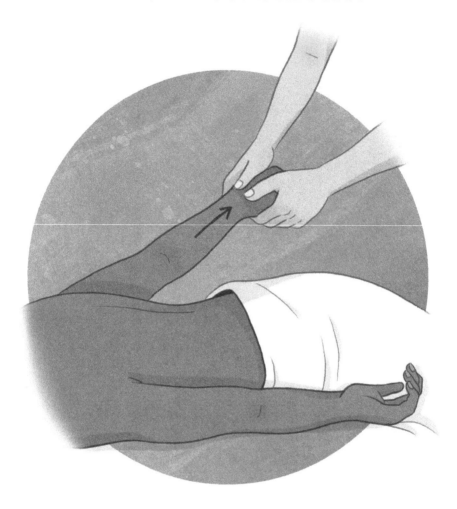

1. Have your partner lie facedown.

2. Pull the arm back, hooking your thumbs between the two bones of the forearm at the elbow.

3. Slide your thumbs down the forearm from the elbow to the wrist to decompress the wrist.

UPPER ARM SQUIGGLES

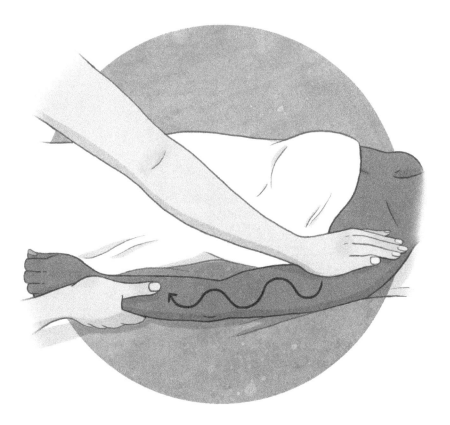

1. With your partner lying faceup, hold their forearm with your wrist.
2. With the other arm, glide down their arm while moving your hand on their forearm back and forward.

DRAINING THE ARM

Use this technique to move stagnant blood flow back up the arms to the torso.

1. Glide the hands up the arm while slowly applying pressure.
2. Repeat this 3 times.

PIN AND STRETCH THE UPPER ARM

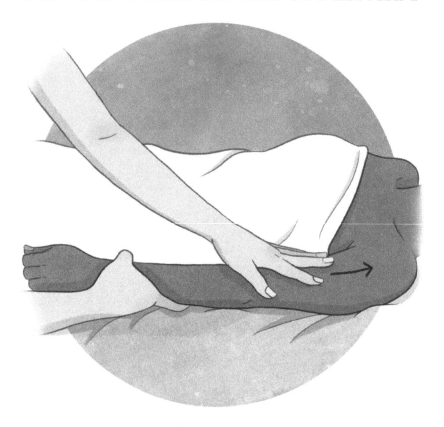

1. Bend the arm at the elbow. Slowly straighten the arm while gliding your hand up the arm toward the body.

2. Repeat to increase range of motion.

SANDWICHING

This technique can be done faceup or facedown.

1. Place one flat palm on the bottom of the arm and one flat palm on top of the arm.

2. Run the top hand along the arm, using the bottom hand for support.

PICK ME UP

This technique helps loosen the forearm and reduce trigger points.

1. Pinch the tissue of the forearm between the thumb and index finger, and roll it gently between your fingers.
2. Hold and compress the tissue if you feel an adhesion or trigger point.

FREE FLOWIN'

This easy arm routine helps create mobility in the arm and shoulder.

1. Use the arm farthest away from your partner to support your partner's wrist.
2. With your other arm, effleurage up the arm from the forearm to the shoulder.
3. Bring the arm out at a 90-degree angle, running your hand back up to the shoulder and back down to their wrist.
4. Bring the arm straight over their head.
5. Glide your hand up the arm to the shoulder and around the armpit into the upper back.
6. Glide the hand back to the wrist. Return the arm to the neutral position.
7. Glide the hand back to the shoulder before moving into the pecs. Repeat on the other arm.

Chest

The chest is primarily composed of the pectoralis major and pectoralis minor muscles. The pecs make up the front of the armpit while the latissimus dorsi makes up the back of the armpit, both attaching on the upper part of the arm. The neck becomes the chest once you dip below the collarbone. The sternum meets at the center of the chest where the ribs branch off. Thoracic outlet syndrome is often the result of tight chest muscles sending numbness and tingling into the arm. For this reason, massaging the chest is a great preventive measure for office workers, desk jockeys, video gamers, artists, and those who read a lot.

PEC PRESS

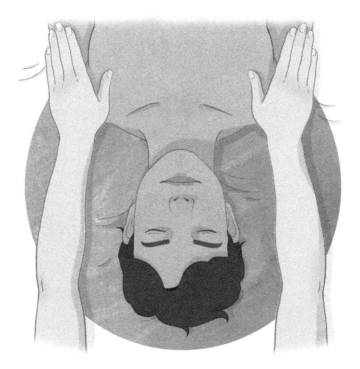

1. Have your partner lie faceup.

2. Press into their chest area gently and hold for 10 to 15 seconds. Then shift your weight from side to side, pressing directly down.

3. Move your hands to the top of each shoulder, and press back and forth with the palm of your hand downward.

PECS AND TWIST

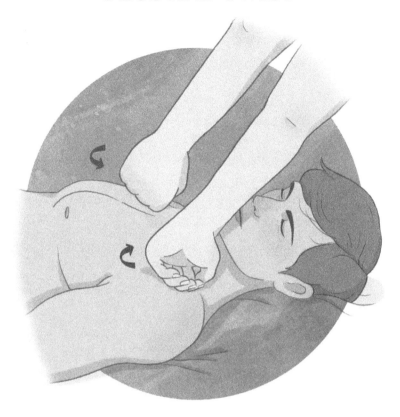

1. Have your partner lie faceup.

2. Make two fists and press each one into your partner's chest while twisting.

3. Gently work your way from the center of the chest to the arm.

CHEST LIFT

This is an easy way to open the chest muscles.

1. Have your partner lie faceup.

2. Sweep your fingertips over the chest. When you reach the armpit, fold the fingers over and lift the pecs of the ribs. Squeeze the pecs and hold for 10 to 15 seconds.

3. Instruct your partner to breathe. Repeat on the other armpit.

ASSISTED PEC STRETCH

1. Have your partner lie on their back. Instruct them to relax their arms.

2. Place one hand on the front of their shoulder. Move the arm up, down, and out while pressing down on the pec.

HOOKED ON YOU

1. With your partner lying facedown, rotate the arm so it falls over the side of your workspace.

2. Loop your arms through their elbow. Move the arm in a circular motion almost as if they were swimming. Then move it in the opposite direction.

3. Repeat with the opposite arm.

RAKING

This technique helps get into the muscles between the ribs.

1. Have your partner lie faceup. Locate the sternum, the bone that runs down the center of the chest. Put your fingertips on either side of it.

2. Rake outward toward the armpits, getting in between the ribs.

INTO THE DEEP

This technique helps get deeper into the chest.

1. Have your partner lie faceup. Bring their arm back over their head, hooking their arm with your arm on the same side.

2. Run your opposite hand down the back of the arm, starting at the elbow, to the chest.

THUMB SCOOPS

1. With your partner lying faceup, locate the collarbone below the neck and above the pecs.

2. Make two fists with your hands. Starting at the center of the chest, rub the tissue of the collarbone, making small "C" motions with your thumbs.

3. Repeat until you reach the armpit.

STACKING HANDS

1. Stand at your partner's side facing them.

2. Locate the sternum in the center of the chest. Place one hand on top of the other over it.

3. Move both hands back toward the armpit in a dragging motion.

Hips and Buttocks

The hips and glutes can be quite burdensome when inflamed. It's often easy to forget that they are responsible for the majority of our movement. Due to sitting, pregnancy, weight gain, and activities that require impact, these areas may often become sore. The buttock is the fleshy area covering the two ischium bones on the back of the body. The two ischia meet at the sacrum where the sciatic nerve comes out between the sacral and lumbar discs. This garden hose–size nerve can be very sensitive when irritated or compressed by muscle, causing pain when moving, sitting, or standing. There are six deep muscles that lie here to help move the hips back and forth, which helps move the leg. The following techniques should be performed with the recipient lying facedown, unless otherwise indicated.

BUNS OF FIRE

This technique can help with lower back pain by stimulating the glute muscles to fire.

1. Plant both of your palms flat on the side of the glute covering the surface.
2. Quickly rock and shake the area.

CARESSING CIRCLES

This technique can help loosen and flush out the gluteal tissue.

Have your partner lie facedown. Flatten your palms and make contact with the glute. Make half circles on the glute, taking one hand over the other when they meet.

GLUTE COMPRESSION

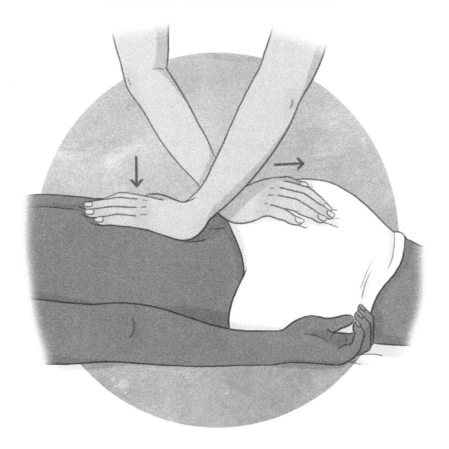

1. Locate where the spine meets the two hip bones at the tailbone and hips.

2. Use your hands to press into the tissue and push in opposite directions. If this hurts your wrists, you may choose to make two fists and begin by gently compressing the area, feeling for areas that are tight. Check in and ask how this feels, because this may be a tender area. If it is tender, do not apply too much pressure, or your recipient may jump off the table.

3. Compress the area and hold. If your hands or wrists become tired, try using an elbow or a knee.

COMPRESS AND SHAKE

This is a great technique to use when you cannot press into the glutes as much as you'd like due to tenderness.

1. Locate areas of tightness in the buttocks by communicating with your partner as you glide your hands over them.

2. Press into the areas of tightness to your partner's comfort level, and shake the area, letting the vibrations help loosen the tissue.

TRIGGER POINT RELIEF FOR GLUTES AND HIP ROTATORS

Use this method to help break up annoying trigger points in the buttocks.

1. Stack the hands and glide off either side of the bone between the hips at the sacrum.

2. Apply friction and circular friction to any areas of tightness to touch.

3. Locate each femur going to the leg and pull the tissue back toward the sacrum.

KNEADED GLUTE RELIEF

Give your partner some "kneaded" relief from sore, overworked glutes with this routine.

1. Petrissage each butt cheek, picking the adhesed tissue up off the muscle.

2. Finish up by flushing the glute tissue out with some light gliding motion and ending with some gentle feathering to soothe the nerves.

3. Repeat on the opposite side.

FREE!

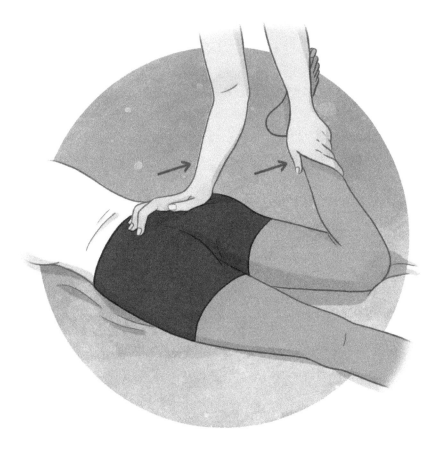

This technique can sometimes free up a nerve in the event that the nerve is impinged by a tight muscle and referring pain to the lower back.

1. Bend the knee 90 degrees, bringing the heel of the foot toward the buttocks.

2. Compress the muscles in the back of the leg below the buttocks but above the knee while lengthening the leg back to the straightened position.

3. Compress areas of tightness in the glute (butt cheek) while rotating the leg to bring the heel of the foot between the same hip and the opposite hip.

4. Straighten the leg and relax it back to the workspace.

5. Flush out the area you have worked with gliding effleurage, and follow it with some light feathering. Compress, shake, and rock the area after.

LOWER BACK AND HIP RELIEF

This orthopedic massage technique is a favorite when dealing with lower back and glute issues.

1. Have the recipient lie faceup.

2. Locate the top of each hip bone. Gently roll your hand over each hip bone, and using the blade of the pinky side of your hand, apply even pressure.

3. Then move your hands to the outside of each hip, facing the recipient, and press into each hip. Have your partner put their hands on your hands and assist you in compressing their hips inward while counting to 20.

4. Have your partner remove their hands. Press downward on each hip, mimicking the way the hips move when you walk, pushing up with one hand and down with the other.

5. Repeat 3 times.

BETTER BUN LIFT

This method releases tension in the buttocks muscles.

1. Start on the outside of the leg where the leg meets the hip.

2. Pick up the tissue from the outside of the leg and hip. Lift the tissue toward the sacrum and the gluteal cleft (yes, the butt crack).

Legs

Reviving tired legs can give you a completely new lease on life. The legs carry the weight of the rest of our body. They are composed of various muscle groups meeting at the hip, knee, and ankle. On the front of the leg below the hip and above the knee, we have the quadriceps group. The back of the leg below the hip and above the knee is the location of the hamstrings. The knee is where the femur, tibia, and fibula meet. The patella is the round knee bone that floats here encased by the quadriceps tendon. Below it you have the shinbone, where people frequently suffer from shin splints when running. On the back of the leg below the knee are the calf muscles.

ROCKING THE LEG

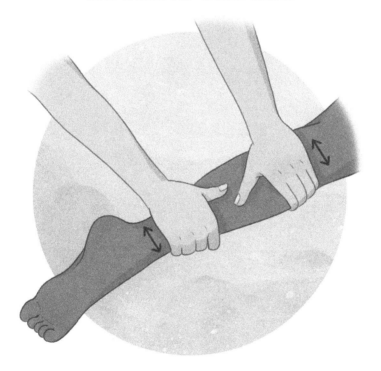

This technique can be done faceup or facedown to help loosen the muscles of the leg without applying pressure.

1. Hook your fingers over the inside of the leg.
2. Push your hands forward and backward to help rock the leg.

TEASING THE TISSUE

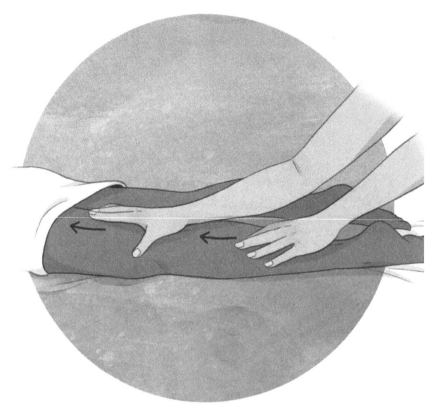

This technique can help improve circulation and flush out the large muscles of the leg and may be done faceup or facedown.

1. Starting at the top of the leg, effleurage upward toward the heart.

2. Repeatedly effleurage in an upward direction, starting a little farther down the leg each time so the strokes get longer and longer.

CIRCULAR KNEE C'S

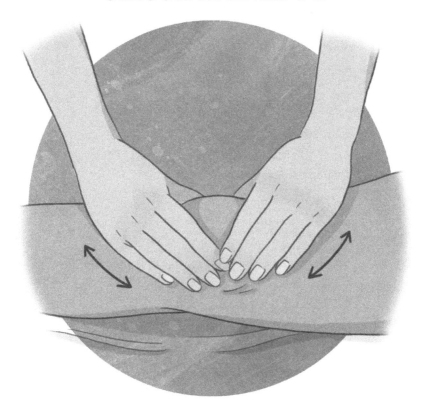

This technique helps create mobility in the knee

1. Form two "C" shapes with your hands.

2. Locate the kneecap and circle around it, squeezing gently. Add in compression and friction as needed.

REVIVING TIRED CALVES

1. Have your partner lie facedown and put the top of their foot on your bent knee.

2. Glide up and down the calf, incorporating petrissage to loosen up the calf muscles.

3. Have your partner point their foot and bring their toes toward their shin. Ask them if they feel any areas of pain or tightness. Revisit areas of discomfort.

4. Glide your hands over the belly of the calf, pushing blood flow back up the leg before ending with light feathering strokes.

PLANTAR RELIEF FOR THE CALVES

1. With your partner lying on their back, glide your hands up the ankle and calf, feeling for areas that may be tight or full.

2. Gently apply steady pressure with the fingertips, or use friction and vibration to help release tension in the area.

3. Feel around the shinbone for areas of muscle that may feel like raisins or bubble wrap, or even make crunching noises. When you locate a spot, gently glide over it repeatedly, compress it with your fingers, or do circular friction until it goes away.

SPREADING THE QUADS

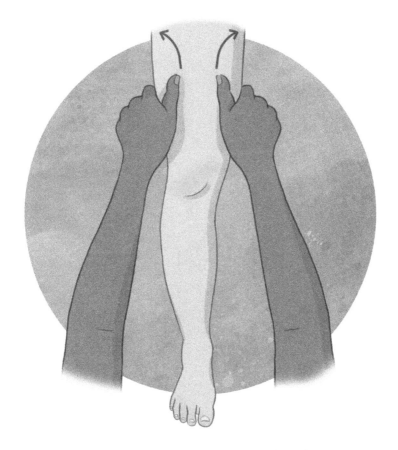

This technique can help relieve knee pain caused by the quadriceps tendon.

1. Have your partner lie faceup.

2. Locate the divot below the knee on the shin where the quadriceps attach. Press to compress the tendon for 10 to 15 seconds before wiggling the kneecap.

3. The side that the kneecap doesn't want to move toward is the tighter part of the quads.

4. Push your fingers and thumbs up the quads, spreading the muscle out and reducing adhesions.

FLUSHING THE QUADRICEPS AND WORKING THE SHIN

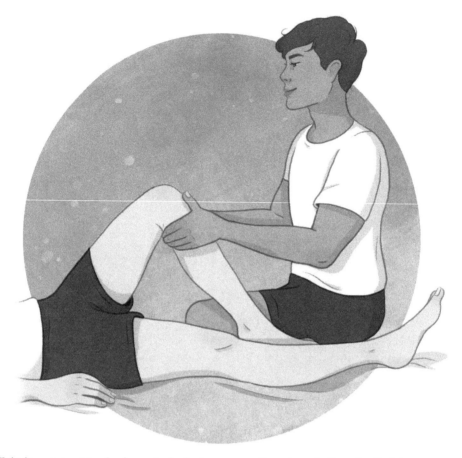

This is a great technique to help improve the circulation in tight quadriceps muscles.

1. Have your partner lie on their back.

2. Bend their knee, keeping the foot planted on your work surface.

3. Sit on their foot to stabilize the leg. Friction the shin with your thumbs, or interlace the fingers and push down the quadriceps muscle from the knee to the hip.

ADDUCTOR RELIEF

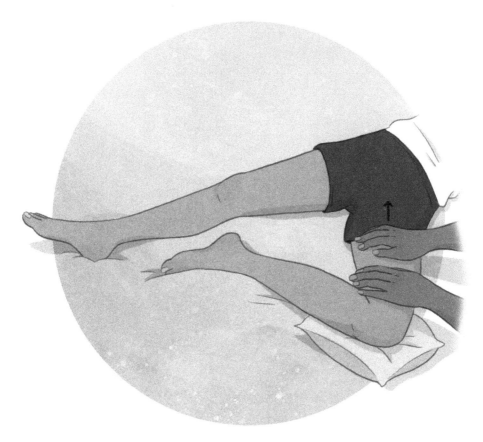

The adductors lie on the inner thigh and may be sensitive to the touch, requiring gentler pressure.

1. Have your partner lie on their back. Bend the knee and rotate the leg out.

2. Gently petrissage the inner thigh.

HAMSTRING HACKING

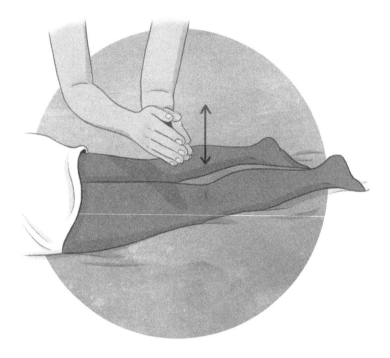

1. Have your partner lie facedown.

2. Flatten your hands and turn them sideways so your palms face each other.

3. Alternately pound them over the hamstrings rapidly.

HAMSTRING COMPRESSIONS

The hamstrings are some of the strongest muscles in the body. Use this technique on stubborn hamstrings.

1. Have your partner lie facedown.

2. Get on your hands and knees. Turn your body perpendicular to your partner's, straddling them so their body is between your hands and knees.

3. Take your shin and press into your partner's hamstrings below the glutes but above the knee. Check in with your partner in regard to pressure.

4. Hold for up to 30 seconds before removing your shin and placing it on another area of the hamstrings.

Feet

The feet are responsible for distributing the weight of your body. They absorb impact when running, walking, or jumping. Without healthy feet, our regular everyday activities are impaired. There are lots of small bones stacked together in the foot. They are surrounded by muscles, tendons, and ligaments. The soles of the feet are the thickest layer of skin in the body. The top of the foot can be sensitive and more tender. One of the biggest issues in feet is plantar fasciitis. This is the inflammation of the fascial layer in the foot. Usually this is due to not wearing shoes with good support, especially for those with high arches.

FOOT MASSAGE FOR ANXIETY

1. Gently glide over the foot, feeling for areas of stress, tension, tightness, or discomfort.

2. Petrissage the instep of the foot.

3. With your thumbs, press into the middle of the foot right below the ball of the foot to activate the acupressure point located there.

4. Next, pinch the area between the big toe and the second toe to compress the acupressure point for anxiety located there, for up to 1 minute.

5. Repeat on the opposite foot.

MASSAGE FOR TRIGGER POINTS OF THE FOOT

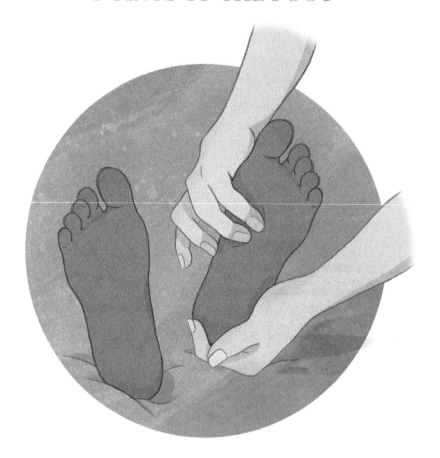

This technique is great for pain specifically in the foot, but may be combined with the technique on page 148 to alleviate symptoms of plantar fasciitis.

1. Begin by gliding over the heel and pad of the foot. Find the arch of the foot, and feel with your fingertips for areas that may be tender or painful. When you find one, hold the spot while checking with your partner on pressure.

2. Apply circular friction to help bring healthy blood flow back to the area.

3. Repeat this over different areas of the foot.

ROCKING FOOT

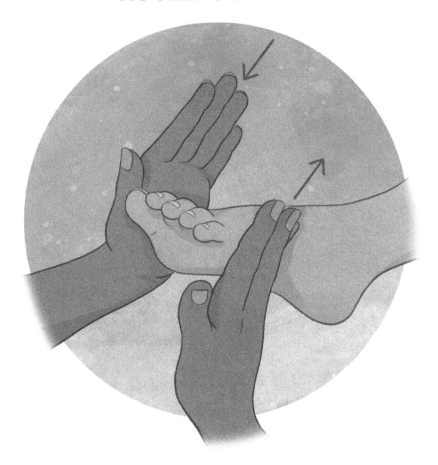

This is a great way to help your partner relax their foot at the beginning of a foot massage, especially if they seem to be stiffening up on you.

1. Gently place the foot loosely between the flat palms of both hands.
2. Move your hands back and forth in opposite directions so the foot moves side to side. Repeat on the other foot.

ARCH ANGEL

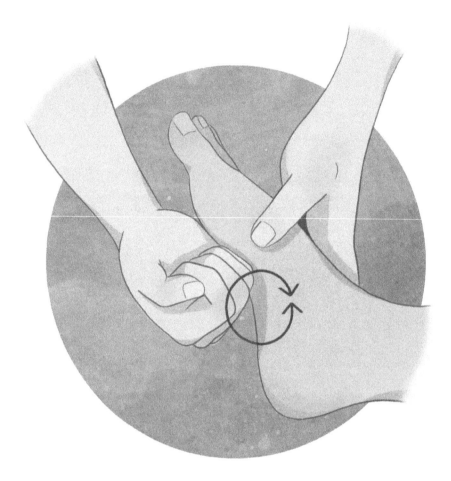

Use this move on your partner if they have high arches in the instep of their foot.

1. Make a fist.

2. Locate the arch of your partner's foot. Push the fist into the foot and rotate. Use your knuckles to help dig into the foot. Repeat on the other foot.

HACKING THE FOOT

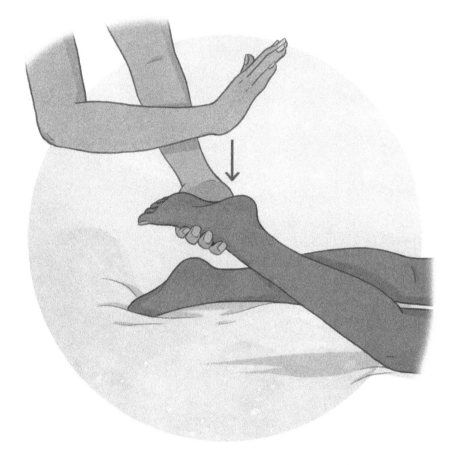

1. With your partner lying facedown, bend the knee to a 45-degree angle.

2. Support the foot with one hand. With the other hand, slap the foot.

3. Repeat with the other foot.

TOE PULLING RELIEF

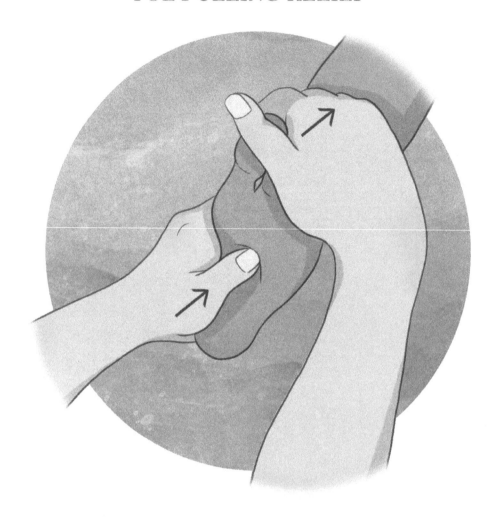

1. Grasp the foot firmly with one hand. Using your other hand, slide your fingers down the big toe, pulling it.

2. Repeat with the remaining four toes and the other foot.

ARCH OPENER

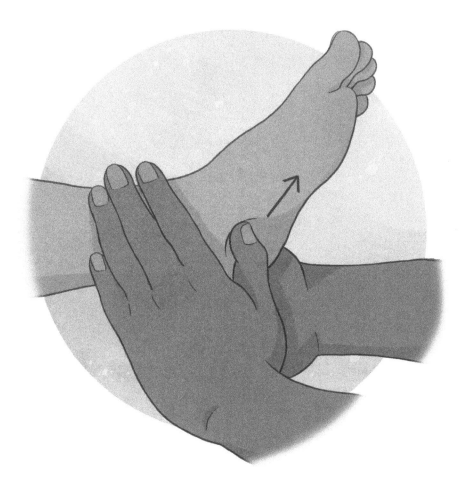

1. Place your hands on either side of the foot with your thumbs parallel on the arch of the foot. Press up into the foot, sliding along the bones of each toe toward the end of the toe with steady, even pressure.

2. Repeat with the other 9 toes.

COMPRESSING THE HEEL

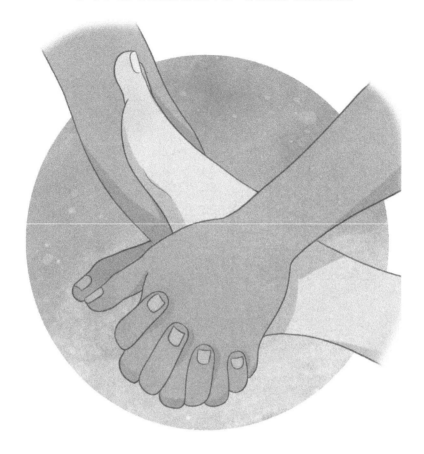

1. Interlace the fingers of both hands and wrap them around the heel, compressing it.

2. From here, you can also rotate the heel and stretch the calf by moving the foot up and down with grasping hands.

GROUNDING THE FEET

Grounding is a way to bring your partner back to the current moment.

1. Sandwich the foot between both hands.

2. Gently rotate the foot and ankle. Flex the foot toward the shin.

3. Extend the foot forward, elongating the top of the foot.

4. Pull both hands off the foot simultaneously. Repeat with the opposite foot.

FOOT FLUSHER

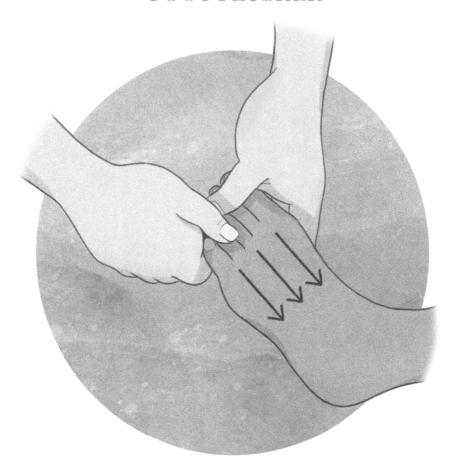

This is a great way to end a foot massage.

1. Starting at the end of each toe below the nail bed, grasp each toe with your thumb and index finger.

2. Glide up toward the ankle with steady pressure following each tendon, pushing blood flow back up the leg.

3. Repeat with the remaining 4 toes.

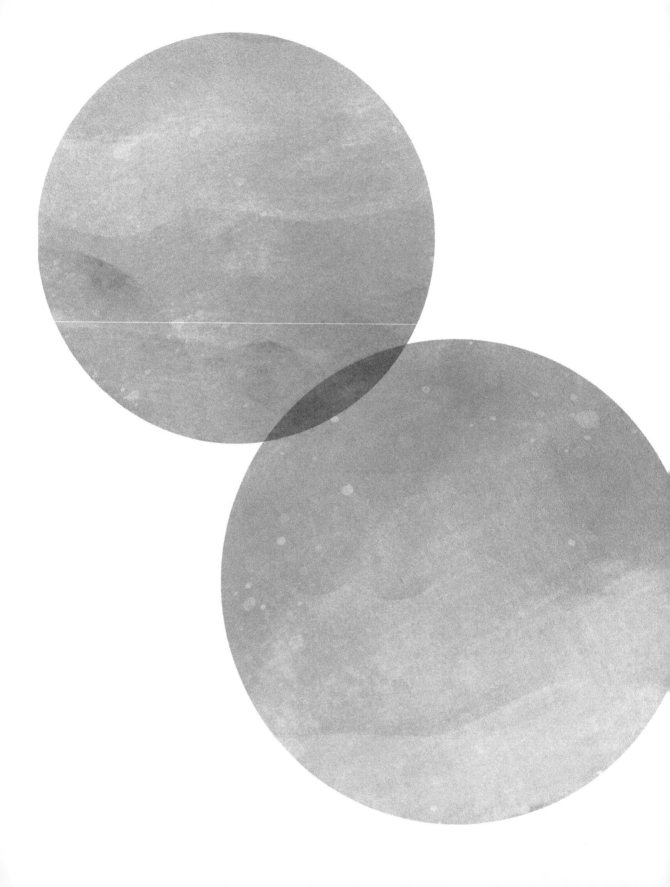

Chapter 7

A Massage for All Reasons

Special occasions require special massages. In this chapter, we will outline massage sequences to help throughout the duration of your relationship. Whether you are experiencing the stress of everyday life, exhaustion from the day-to-day routine, or a new addition to the family, these massage sequences are here for you to adapt and make your own in the comfort of your home. The more comfortable you get and the more you practice at home, the more confidence you will feel when massaging your partner.

TENSION TAMER

Life can be stressful. The goal of the Tension Tamer is to help relax after a stressful day at work or when uncomfortable events attempt to seize hold of your relationship with your partner. Use this massage to keep the anxiety from work or play at bay. Mix 4 drops of lavender, 4 drops of bergamot, and 4 drops of sweet orange per 1 ounce of carrier oil, or diffuse in a diffuser to provide a tension-taming scent.

1. Start with your partner facedown, using some long, slow, relaxing effleurage. Then massage one side at a time, rocking and shaking into the lats.

2. Hold areas that are tense with broad, even pressure from the palm or forearm while encouraging your partner to breathe.

3. Massage small circles around the palms of the hands. Rake your hands up the arms toward the shoulder. Squeeze the shoulders before doing some frictioning down the neck.

4. End with a nice scalp massage using the fingertips and the knuckles.

FATIGUE FIGHTER

We all get tired sometimes. This is a great massage to start the day or at midday when you want to crash but can't. Make a special essential oil concoction with 6 drops of lime and 6 drops of lemon in a carrier oil like jojoba.

1. Begin with a stimulating scalp massage with hair tugging.

2. Move to the face and try the EFT Tapping technique (page 100) to help with fatigue and focus.

3. Massage the ears to energize the mood.

4. Next, have your partner lie on their stomach and give a vigorous back and neck massage with lots of rocking and shaking.

5. Do some tapotement on the back. Stretch the legs and the arms.

APHRODISIAC

Perhaps your partner needs a little help forgetting the rest of the world and focusing on pleasure. Mix 4 drops of bergamot, 3 drops of orange, 2 drops of coriander, 2 drops of ylang ylang, 1 drop of geranium, and 1 drop of jasmine in 1 ounce of carrier oil such as jojoba or coconut to use during this massage, if your partner desires.

1. Have your partner lie facedown.

2. Gently massage the back, focusing on the area around the spine and lower back. Perform effleurage and waves on the lower back.

3. Move into the gluteal area, doing some circling.

4. Have your partner roll over.

5. Massage the nape of the neck using some circular friction where the base of the head meets the neck. Massage the face and scalp, paying special attention to the midline, using effleurage and even light tapping. Massage the abdomen with some gentle circles going in a clockwise motion.

6. End with a foot massage, paying special attention to the instep.

IMMUNE BOOST

Use this massage when one of you starts to feel a little sickly. It's an immune system pick-me-up. An essential oil blend made with eucalyptus will help open up the nasal passages in the event of congestion. Add 6 drops of lavender and 6 drops of eucalyptus essential oil per 1 ounce of carrier oil such as coconut.

1. Start with your partner faceup. Instruct them to take a few deep breaths to inhale the essential oil mixture as you hold it over their nose.

2. Start with the face. Sweep your fingers down either side of the nose toward the corners of the mouth 3 times. Then pinch the inner eyebrows to help relieve the sinuses before running both hands outward from the center of the top lip to the jaw. Gently tug the earlobes and massage tiny circles behind the ears. Glide the hands down the neck. Effleurage the chest, pushing all blood flow back to the lymph nodes.

3. Effleurage down their arms, gently rubbing small circles along the joints of the hands. Pay special attention to the reflex points for the sinuses lying in the fingertips.

4. Next, have your partner expose their abdomen. Using a lotion or essential oil mixture, gently glide your hands over the abdomen in a clockwise motion going in the direction of the colon. Be aware that the aorta also lies here, so if you feel a pulse, back off.

5. You may choose to gently lift under the back, coming back to the abdomen, getting as close as possible to where the spine meets the hip bones.

6. Flush the abdomen using a gliding motion counterclockwise back over the abdomen, fading into a feathered stroke. Effleurage down the legs, starting with short strokes pushing back toward the groin.

7. Grasp one foot. Gently bend the toes. Perform circular friction on the tips of the toes where the reflexology points are for the sinuses. Repeat on the other foot.

8. Have your partner roll over. Gently effleurage the back, pushing blood flow toward the lymph nodes in the armpits. Perform some tapotement on the back such as cupping.

9. End with a feathered stroke.

SWEET DREAMS

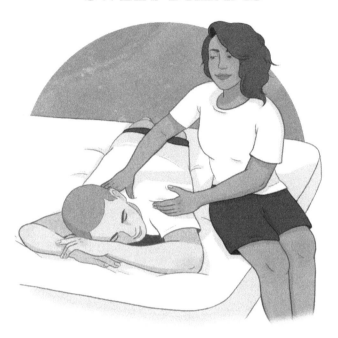

Getting deep, beautiful, restful sleep is important for both of you. Helping each other wind down and ease into a slumber can become a relaxing ritual. I recommend trading off so that one person receives a bedtime massage one night and the other receives it the next night. That way, you both get a chance to drift off to sleep directly after your massage. Consider adding lavender to your lotion for a better night's slumber.

1. Start with your partner facedown.

2. Move to one side of the body, and petrissage the sides. Gently friction the neck and the shoulders, combining in effleurage.

3. Work down the arms using effleurage and petrissage.

4. When you reach the hands, gently friction and compress the joints. Now start focusing on one hand. Stretch the fingers by bending the joints. Effleurage back up the arm, pushing blood flow back toward the heart. Repeat on the other arm.

CONTINUES

5. Next, compress the glutes. If your partner is comfortable, you can effleurage and petrissage them; however, this can be an emotionally charged area, like the inner thighs. Move to the back of the leg, using effleurage to warm up the tissue and apply the lubricant. Use a fist, hand, or forearm to friction or compress the back of the thigh before moving on to petrissage the back of the thigh. Use effleurage to provide a transition from the thigh to the calf, working in petrissage and friction.

6. Move to the foot, using fiction and circular friction to increase the circulation to the foot. If you find anything in the foot that feels hard or crunchy, compress it for 10 to 15 seconds. Gently stretch and bend the toes, frictioning each joint. Move back to the ankle, using longer effleurage strokes to push the flow of blood back up the leg. Move to the other side of the body. Repeat, starting at the beginning of step 5.

7. Have your partner turn over so they are faceup. Compress the shoulders using light effleurage and friction over the chest from the armpits up, before moving to the arm. Do the same motions down the arms to the fingers, ending with focusing on the small joints. Move back up the arm, using effleurage to push blood flow back to the body. Repeat on the other arm.

8. Next, we are going to start effleurage and petrissage on one of your partner's legs, adding friction in a circular motion around the kneecap. Effleurage the front of the calf, using both hands to glide up and down both sides of the shinbone. Create friction on the foot, getting in between the small bones. Use effleurage to assist the blood flow back up the leg. Repeat on the other leg.

9. Go back to the head and neck. Use effleurage to apply lotion to both areas. Friction the muscles of the neck down the face toward the body. Compress areas of tightness using your hands and fingers.

10. Move to the face. Glide hands over the cheeks with small light strokes 3 times. Then glide each hand from the nose out to the cheek 3 times. Then move to the forehead, making small light circles over the temples before doing sweeping effleurage from the center of the forehead to the neck. Gently compress the forehead before using your fingertips all at once to do circular friction on the scalp. Slow down with your circles until you come to a stop.

PMS SOOTHER

Premenstrual syndrome, with symptoms like cramps and mood swings, can be a sore spot in the month for partners. The monthly shift of hormones can also cause acne, lower back pain, headaches, joint pain, bloating, and abdominal cramping. Use this technique to slay the PMS monster regardless of whether you are giving or receiving this wonderful massage. The use of warm rice packs that can be reheated in the microwave or warm wet towels warmed up with an essential oil such as geranium or bergamot can be a nice addition during this time as well.

1. Instruct your recipient to lie faceup. If you wish, you may begin with some light face and scalp massage to help move the lymph system, which may be slower due to bloating and swelling.

2. Hook your hands under the base of the skull in the parallel hollow areas between the two vertical neck muscles. Hold to stimulate the Gates of Consciousness, the pressure points known to regulate menstrual cramps. Move your hands to 1 inch under the big bump at the bottom of the skull, and then move your hands out a few inches into the hollows between the muscles on the back of the neck.

3. Perform small circles at the base of the head to loosen and help with any PMS-related headaches.

4. Massage the hands, paying extra attention to the back of the hand just above the wrist bones where the reflexology points for the female reproductive organs are found.

5. Remove sheets or clothing from the abdomen. Apply oil or lotion to the abdomen. Locate your partner's lower left abdominal quadrant. Use friction to create small circles sweeping downward to loosen the contents and move the contents further through the intestines, moving any gas bubbles and breaking up hardened fecal matter making it hard to eliminate. After every couple of circles, move upward, followed by a downward feathering motion, sweeping everything back toward the rectum. Once you reach right below the rib cage, move horizontally to the right, still following the same circular pattern.

CONTINUES

6. Once you reach the right upper quadrant under the ribs, move downward with circular friction while continuing to move everything around and out of the large intestines. When you get to the lower right quadrant above the hip bone, you may notice more tenderness and need to work lighter, but continue with gentle circular friction.

7. Locate the belly button, and stimulate the spot about three fingers below the navel, known as the Sea of Energy acupressure point, for up to 1 minute. Then locate the Gate Origin point, four fingers below the belly button, and continue to apply circular friction to the area.

8. Glide your hands gently up and down the hip bones, locating the crease between the legs and abdomen in the groin. You do not want to use heavy pressure due to lymph nodes, arteries, and veins being located here. Several acupressure points are located here, which would benefit from small circles and light effleurage to help with bloating, constipation, and pain down the legs.

9. Use gentle effleurage down the legs to help soothe ligament pain. Massage the feet, paying special attention to where the arches and the outer and inner ankle are located, as that's where the female organ system lives in reflexology.

10. Have your partner roll over onto their abdomen so they are facedown. Begin with the calves and legs, using light effleurage to soothe ligament pains and help move fluid.

11. Next, move to the glutes. There are quite a few acupressure points located in the glutes and lower back related to PMS. Perform some compressions using your fists. Pushing into the glute and rocking can help loosen tight muscles, activate the acupressure points, and help relieve lower back pain.

12. Move to the back to perform some long, soothing effleurage strokes before moving into some petrissage on the lower back.

13. End with some petrissage on the shoulders to help activate the shoulder-well points, which can help with PMS.

PREGNANCY

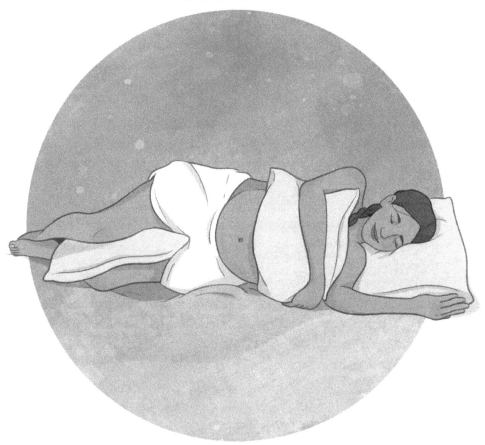

Pregnancy can be taxing on the mind and body. There are many changes happening physically, mentally, emotionally, and hormonally as your family grows. Prenatal massage is a great way to support your partner in the preparation for birth. Although I do not recommend massage during the first trimester, massage later in the pregnancy can do wonders to soothe the nerves as well as the whole body. After 12 weeks, when hormones have begun to stabilize and the fetus has firmly implanted, massage is a great way to help the mom-to-be.

CONTINUES

PREGNANCY *continued*

For this massage, you will need a flat surface and multiple pillows to use as props. A stool is optional for sitting versus standing. If your partner is uncomfortable lying down, she may sit in a chair. Light to medium pressure is advised. Compressions should not be held for more than 10 to 15 seconds maximum, and no area should be focused on too heavily. Avoid heavy pressure of any kind on the legs—particularly the inner legs—as blood volume doubles during pregnancy and the body begins to produce more clotting factors to prepare for childbirth. Typically, percussive methods such as hacking or cupping should be avoided during pregnancy. Induction points can be stimulated after week 38 and are in the feet and ankles; however, the feet and ankles can still be massaged gently. In the event that she has significant puffiness or swelling, ask a doctor before proceeding with massage.

1. Have your partner lie on her side on a flat surface such as the bed or couch.

2. Place a pillow under the head and neck. You may wish to bunch the pillow closest to the shoulder to fill the space next to the neck for further comfort. Have them straighten their bottom leg and bend their top leg. Stack pillows under the bent top leg until the leg is parallel to the surface they are lying on.

3. A towel may be placed under the belly to prevent the strain of intrauterine ligaments if she feels as if she's falling or being pulled forward. A pillow may be hugged to the chest to support the arm.

4. Begin by placing a hand on the shoulder and the side of the head. Gently push into the shoulder to stretch the neck. Effleurage, friction, and petrissage the neck area. Prior to 38 weeks avoid compressing any point or working on it for too long during the massage.

5. Move on to the shoulders and back. The use of a stool may provide some support with body mechanics but is not required. Stretch the lats by crossing your arms and gently pressing and rocking the side of the body. Great techniques to use on the back include circling, effleurage, and petrissage. Gentle friction along the spine and hips may be nice for new mothers struggling with back pain. Pay special attention to the lower back, as many expectant mothers struggle with the weight of the baby pushing the hips outward, causing strain on the area.

6. Optionally, you may lightly effleurage the abdomen. This may feel especially wonderful around the hips due to the strain on ligaments. Never use heavy pressure over the abdomen, as it could potentially be dangerous for the baby. However, abdominal massage can potentially help with stretch marks by increasing circulation.

7. Gently compress the glutes using your fists. The Twisty Fists technique may be a nice way to help reduce pain and fatigue in this area. Next, massage the leg area. Avoid the inner thigh, and always use light pressure on the legs with strokes moving upward toward the body to assist with improving blood flow, avoiding clots, and reducing swelling. Never perform massage on your partner if a dent appears when you press into the tissue. If this happens, immediately follow up with your doctor. Fullness in the hands, feet, and ankles may occur due to the weight and pressure of the baby, as well as blood volume, but massage is safe when approved by a doctor. Raking and light effleurage are great movements during this time.

8. Pregnant women love to have their feet massaged. Avoid heavy pressure and compression on points of the feet before 38 weeks, as these may cause preterm labor. Direct all strokes back up toward the torso.

9. Repeat on the opposite side of the body.

Resources

American Massage Therapy Association (AMTA) and Associated Bodywork and Massage Professionals (ABMP)
Follow the AMTA and the AMBP for new research and developments on the benefits of massage and to get more information on how to pursue a career in the massage field. Visit them online at AMTAmassage.org and ABMP.com for more details.

Badass Bodyworkers
Visit BadassBodyworkers.com for a list of the best massage and bodywork therapists across the United States, including those who offer professional couples massage and couples massage courses near you.

Chopra Center
Visit Chopra.com for more on Ayurvedic traditions and to take their dosha assessment.

Perfect Pockets Plus
Check out PerfectPocketsPlus.com for a wide variety of hot and cold packs and holsters for lotion.

Pro Health Systems
Visit ProHealthSys.com to learn more about massage, botanical medicine, yoga, and how to improve the way the body moves from Dr. Nikita Vizniak, and continue learning about the body with books, seminars, and tools.

Robert Gardner Wellness
Visit RobertGardnerWellness.com for books, DVDs, and at-home workbooks. Subscribe to the Thai massage subscription service for $7 per month to learn Thai Yoga Massage in the comfort of your home.

Simply Earth

Visit SimplyEarth.com for all your essential oil and massage oil needs. You'll feel good knowing they send 13 percent of their profits every month to benefit a different organization fighting human trafficking.

Universal Coach Institute

The Universal Coach Institute supplies quality coaching instruction for future coaches, offering programs in life coaching, business coaching, and relationship coaching. Visit UniversalCoachInstitute.org for more information or to find a certified relationship coach and enhance the closeness of your relationship with your significant other.

References

Bleecker, Deborah. *Acupuncture Points Handbook*. Dallas: Draycott Publishing, 2017.

———. *Acupressure Made Simple*. Dallas: Draycott Publishing, 2019.

Cohen, Don. *An Introduction to Craniosacral Therapy*. Berkeley, Calif.: North Atlantic Books, 1995.

Kunz, Barbara, and Kevin Kunz. *Complete Reflexology for Life*. New York: Dorling Kindersley, 2009.

———. *Reflexology: Health at Your Fingertips*. New York: Dorling Kindersley Publishing, 2016.

Lundberg, Paul. *The New Book of Shiatsu*. London: Octopus Publishing Group, 2014.

Steele, Cindy. *Tantric Massage*. Self-published, 2015.

Weis-Bohlen, Susan. *Ayurveda Beginner's Guide*. Emeryville, Calif.: Althea Press, 2018.

Index

Acknowledgments

I would like to thank the fabulous team at Callisto for this opportunity, particularly my editor, Rochelle Torke, for her direction. I would like to thank my staff for all their patience with me while I worked on this book. Katherine Stevenson did an amazing job managing everyone at the office and was crucial in making this book possible. Thank you to my eight-year-old, Skyler, for understanding that Mommy had to write. I pray that you grow up to learn the power of consent and healthy touch. A shout-out to my parents for watching Skyler for multiple weekends and giving me the peace and quiet so that I could write. A big thank-you to my clients for understanding that I was having to temporarily reorganize my life to make this book come to life. My friends and colleagues—Michelle Holleman, Shilah Roethel, Rebecca Brumfield, Robert Gardner, Laura Allen, Amber Love, and the Spapreneurs—for all your great advice and support and for keeping me on track as well as answering my random questions without a second thought. Thank you, Laura Tompkins and Kariann Ross with Laurel Belle Photography, as well as Michele Whaley for making me beautiful and dressing me for promotional photos. I couldn't have done it without you. Thank you all for all your love and support!

About the Author

ASHLEY DWYER, LMT (NC LMBT #14844), is a licensed massage and bodywork therapist in Charlotte, North Carolina. She spends most of her days massaging clients at her practice, Fire & Ice Therapeutic Massage. When she is not there, she is busy developing new courses and teaching continuing education classes for massage therapists at the Massage Innovation Network for Therapists, consulting for small businesses, and practicing life, business, and relationship coaching. In her free time, she enjoys hiking (particularly near waterfalls) and camping with her son, Skyler, traveling, and snuggling with their two cats.